Psychological Consultation With a Police Department

A Report Submitted to

The Hogg Foundation for Mental Health

Will C. Hogg Building
University of Texas
Austin, Texas

Psychological Consultation With A Police Department

A DEMONSTRATION OF COOPERATIVE TRAINING IN MENTAL HEALTH

By

PHILIP A. MANN, Ph.D.

Associate Professor of Psychology
Indiana University
Bloomington, Indiana

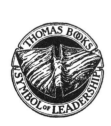

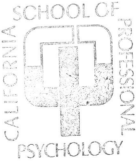

CHARLES C THOMAS · PUBLISHER

Springfield · Illinois · U.S.A.

Published and Distributed Throughout the World by
CHARLES C THOMAS • PUBLISHER
BANNERSTONE HOUSE
301-327 East Lawrence Avenue, Springfield, Illinois, U.S.A.

© *1973, by* CHARLES C THOMAS • PUBLISHER

ISBN-0-398-02695-5

Library of Congress Catalog Card Number: 72-88486

With THOMAS BOOKS *careful attention is given to all details of manufacturing and design. It is the Publisher's desire to present books that are satisfactory as to their physical qualities and artistic possibilities and appropriate for their particular use.* THOMAS BOOKS *will be true to those laws of quality that assure a good name and good will.*

Printed in the United States of America
C-1

INTRODUCTION

THE FREQUENCY with which the police have been a leading subject of study of the several Presidential Commissions during
the 1960's provides striking evidence of the character of the times,
of society's views of itself, and of the police, and of the often conflicting responsibilities which are assigned to this major institution.
Alongside of this evidence, it is even more remarkable that policemen as a group are so isolated from most of society and so little
known and understood by the citizenry. One could hardly imagine
a situation better designed to create misunderstanding and controversy.

Society assigns to the police responsibilities for maintaining
safety, security, and order, while the model citizen behaves toward
the police as though he believed that "what you don't know can't
hurt you." The normal social goal in relationships with the police,
for both criminals and non-criminals, is to avoid contact. In addition to serving as a reassurance of innocence, this attitude also
reflects the fact that society expects policemen to deal with problems and people with whom it, as a group, wishes to avoid contact.

Yet, there is another aspect of police work which is all too often
obscured by this dominant social relationship to the police. For
some people, frequently but not always a part of the population
defined by lower rank in social and economic characteristics, the
police constitute the most readily available and logical resource
for help with human problems. Historically, the police were for
some people a familiar source of guidance, friendship, and a
readily accessible representative of community authority in the
positive sense of the term. Today some policemen still carry and
cherish that image of themselves in their relations with certain
aspects of community life. Changes in social complexity, and effi-

ciency measures which have changed the organization of police work have greatly diminished this feature of the policeman's job.

But, whether nostalgic or not, policemen today are still called upon to provide service to people with problems with greater relative frequency than they are required to intervene in criminal matters. Most police administrators and officers recognize this; regardless of their liking for the assignment, most of them realize the importance of handling such assignments well; but few citizens are aware of the policeman's contribution to this phase of community life, and the policeman is seldom rewarded for his performance of these tasks.

Another development of the 1960's, the community mental health movement, recognized the importance of this part of police work, along with the contributions of other persons who, unofficially and without professional training, contributed to the mental health efforts of the community. These persons, who in the professional terminology of the field are referred to as *natural caregivers,* were seen early as logical allies in attempting to improve the mental health of the community. By providing consultative services to improve the help-giving efforts of these caregivers, the goal is to make more widely effective use of the skills of professionally trained mental health personnel than could be accomplished by their conducting direct treatment services, and to reach populations who have traditionally underused the official mental health resources. The emphasis in this movement is on the achievement of preventive goals through increased reliance on agents to whom many people normally turn in attempting to deal with their problems in living.

This report describes one program, which is part of the developing activities in the field of community mental health, wherein a group of psychologists provided consultative services to the police department in Austin, Texas. In keeping with the demonstration character of the project, this report is written in the hope of stimulating other communities to conduct similar programs and to provide the benefits of this experience in their efforts to do so.

In the Fall of 1969, the Hogg Foundation for Mental Health awarded a grant to the Austin Police Department to conduct a two-year demonstration project in psychological consultation. This project was the product of far-sighted leadership in both the Austin Police Department and the Hogg Foundation, and came to fruition through discussion and clarification of the mutual goals of these two institutions. It was this kind of beginning that made the project possible.

The project was conceived from its origin as one which could be beneficial to the community through providing helpful experiences for policemen and for the graduate students in community psychology at the University of Texas who were to participate in it. In the following pages the project is described, along with its rationale and activities, and an attempt is made to evaluate its successes and limitations in order that some of the methods employed might be improved upon and/or adopted for use in other communities.

The author of this report has served as the supervising consultant for the project, and while the style and content emerge necessarily from his own conceptual framework, the preparation of this report has been accompanied by constant reminders of the contributions of numerous individuals whose theoretical and practical suggestions, as well as hard work, have been instrumental in conducting the activities described here. In addition to Chief Robert Miles and the entire Austin Police Department, special acknowledgment is due to former police Captain J. C. Fann and Captain Don Doyle for their help in the original planning of this project, to Assistant Chief George Phifer and Majors B. F. Rosen and Benny McDavid for their help and encouragement in coordinating various activities, and in particular to Captain Harland Moore who provided virtual daily coordination of the project in the form of making introductions, interpreting the project to policemen, and serving as an invaluable source of information and advice, while at the same time carrying on a heavy load of police-community relations responsibilities.

Dr. Robert Sutherland, former president; Dr. Wayne Holtzman, president; and Col. Stanley Brown, Assistant for Administration, of the Hogg Foundation provided wise counsel as well as encouragement throughout the project. Dr. Ira Iscoe, Director of the Community Mental Health Training Program at the University of Texas was especially helpful in his encouragement and suggestions, as well as in providing support through his relationships in the community.

The graduate students who participated in the project were Kim Hamblin, David Hopkinson, Kenneth Kopel, William Levin, Dennis Lindorfer, and Thomas Tudor. Their work as consultants, trainers and researchers was indispensable to the project, and it can only be hoped that the experience they gained can partially repay their efforts.

Finally, special thanks are due to Barrett Alexander, who served as research assistant to the project, and to Patty Cox and Janet Peckinpaugh who provided secretarial services.

PHILIP A. MANN

To Jane, Marci, and Jon

CONTENTS

Psychological Consultation With a Police Department

PART I

BACKGROUND

Chapter I

POLICE FUNCTIONS AND MENTAL HEALTH STRATEGIES

R ESEARCH OVER THE PAST two decades has highlighted the gulf between the dimensions of mental health problems in the United States and the extent and effectiveness of programs aimed at their solution (Joint Commission on Mental Illness and Health, 1961). Efforts to alleviate this problem have led to a number of innovative programs under the impetus of the community mental health movement (Cowen, Gardner and Zax, 1967).

While the literature is becoming increasingly diverse and voluminous, some central features of the problem can be cited which are particularly salient to mental health program planning. First, mental illness is expensive. The more conservative estimates suggest that about ten percent of the population is in need of formal mental health services, with some estimates running as high as one-third of the population (Cowen, Gardner and Zax, 1967, pp. 14-15). While exact costs of the problem are difficult to calculate, if one considers that costs range from $4,000 to process an adolescent through a juvenile court system to nearly a quarter of a million dollars for lifetime hospitalization of a psychotic patient (Cowen, Gardner and Zax, 1967, p. 416), the cost is staggering by any yardstick.

Second, only a minority of those who admit they could use help with a mental health problem actually seek professional services (Gurin, Veroff and Feld, 1960) and those who are seen by professional mental health practitioners may not be those in greatest need (Hollingshead and Redlich, 1958).

Third, even with this restriction in the use of services, the supply of professional manpower is hopelessly inadequate to meet the demand of those who do seek services (Albee, 1959). At the

5

same time, there is evidence that people do seek help with mental health problems from a number of nonmental health sources who they see as more appropriate and/or accessible than the official mental health agents (Gurin, Veroff and Feld, 1960; Kelly, 1964).

These and other considerations have led to a change in orientation from the study of the etiology and dynamics of the individual case to an examination of incidence and prevalence rates in population as a consequence of cultural and social conditions, and a change in emphasis from intensive dyadic treatment methods to preventive strategies and the enhancement of positive effectiveness in living (Caplan, 1964), for many workers in the mental health field.

Some preventive strategies attempt to capitalize on crisis situations which provide an opportunity for growth as well as a threat to mental health (Caplan, 1961). A central focus of these preventive interventions are the natural caregivers in communities who are already in contact with persons in need of help. Often, such persons are in a more advantageous position to implement crisis intervention measures than are official mental health agents by virtue of the fact that since they are more visible and have a more continuous relationship with persons in need, they are more likely to be sought out in times of crisis.

The Police as a Caregiving Group

The urban police department is a significant mental health agency. Despite the fact that its status as such is seldom recognized by the public, by mental health professionals, or the police themselves, the research of Hollingshead and Redlich (1958), Cumming, Cumming and Edell (1965), and Liberman (1969) has substantiated the significance of the policeman's role in mental health, particularly in bringing lower class patients to treatment.

The other side of the coin, similarly little known, is that mental health problems play a large role in the police field, in both numbers and importance. In urban police departments, requests for assistance with family crises make up about half the calls which the police receive, other than traffic cases. Furthermore, these calls are among the most dangerous missions which policemen undertake. Over twenty percent of police fatalities in the line of duty, and about forty percent of the line of duty injuries, occur while responding to such calls (Bard, 1969a).

There is typically a glaring discrepancy between the activity of the policeman in this area and the limited training he has had in behavioral science and human relations. Perhaps some of this discrepancy is due to the widely held belief that police work should deal only with criminal activity and that policemen should not be social workers. However, this belief is rapidly changing throughout the country, as the human relations problems facing policemen become more obvious and critical, and as the functions of police departments as behavior mediating institutions become clearer. Rather than becoming social workers, policemen are seeking to become more effective representatives of the community in times of human trouble.

Impetus for professionals to work closely with police comes from several sources. Programs such as the Houston police-community human relations training project have arisen directly from the crisis in race relations (Sikes and Cleveland, 1968). As the concept of community mental health develops, the police department is becoming an important locus of intervention for preventive programs (Bard and Berkowitz, 1967; Mann, 1971). The police themselves have recognized the need to increase the training which policemen receive not only to improve their effectiveness, but also in order to recruit and retain better qualified personnel through upgrading the standards of the police profession.

Within the perspective of community mental health, the police department is in a unique position to implement preventive programs in the course of their regular work. Most police work with citizens occurs in the context of crisis, a time believed to be especially ripe for behavioral change (Rapoport, 1962). In many family crises to which the police are called, the mere presence of the police serves to restore a temporary family equilibrium. Appropriate action on their part could serve to forestall future crises, arrange for referrals for more extended help, or help to prevent injury or death to family members.

Furthermore, the police are one of the few community agencies which is in operation 24-hours-a-day, every day. The mental health problems which they encounter are highly likely to be those which are not presented to the usual mental health-oriented community agencies, and they are in contact with populations which do not ordinarily avail themselves of traditional services.

As a result, the policeman is often the mental health agent of last resort for some persons. Among these are the poor, who then become over-represented among state hospital populations, and those whose mental health problems deviate from the legal and social norms of the community in ways that make it difficult for them to obtain treatment without incrimination or ostracism; the drug user, alcoholic and sexual deviate. When the delinquent, ambulatory psychotic and compulsive criminal are added to the list, the mental health role of the policeman looms large in comparison to the usual treatment population of the trained mental health professional (Hollingshead and Redlich, 1958).

But the importance of behavioral science training for policemen does not end here. The majority of the policeman's activities involve delicate human relations, whether in dealing with persons from different ethnic and cultural backgrounds from his own, or presenting a traffic citation to a middle class person with a strong *law-abiding* self-image. Through experience, policemen learn to become sensitive observers of human behavior. Training does not need to be directed towards increasing this sensitivity, but rather to the interpretation of and appropriate response to the cues which the policeman observes but may not know how to use.

A second training need which police have frequently is in establishing cooperation with community agencies as sources of mutual support and referral. Part of the problem is a lack of information, but there are also such factors as a tendency to protect the *territory* of each institution on the part of police and agency personnel, and a desire on both sides to avoid the *negative image* of the other. The police do not wish to be seen as social workers; agency workers prefer not to be authority figures. Yet, where police and agency workers have an opportunity to become acquainted on a face-to-face basis, cooperation can be increased and the effectiveness of both institutions improved.

History of the Project

The Austin Police Department has recognized the need for improving its training program and the educational level of the police force. A number of workshops and training sessions have been conducted in recent years. A *Buddy System* in which citizens ride with policemen to become better acquainted with police activities has been successfully implemented. Students from the University of Texas Law School have also been involved in the Buddy System, as well as in research using police department records to increase their understanding of police work.

In the fall of 1968, the Austin Police Department arranged through the Extension Division of the University of Texas to offer a course in basic psychology for policemen. This course succeeded in giving policemen a better understanding of human behavior, and furthered the process of stimulating an interest among policemen in continuing education (Mann, 1970). After completing the course in psychology, several individual officers have enrolled in other university courses, and arrangements have been made with nearby colleges to provide more complete police science curricula.

Another outcome of the psychology course was a recognition by many policemen that they would benefit more from continuous training in the application of psychological principles to their everyday activities. Discussions with members of the police department established the need for this further training and suggested the consultant model as the most workable one. In the remainder of this chapter, the rationale of the project is described. Activities which implemented these plans are described in subsequent chapters.

DESIGN OF THE PROJECT
Psychological Consultation

Consultation is a mutually cooperative problem-solving process between consultant and consultee. It is limited to the contribution which the consultant can make from his sphere of expertise to the work-role related problems which the consultee presents (Rhodes, 1960). This model seems to lend itself well to a continuous in-service training program.

From the consultant's standpoint, consultation makes wider use of the consultant's professional skills through collaboration with consultees who can reach a larger number of clients than the professional himself could contact individually, and who are in contact with persons unlikely to seek the services of a mental health professional initially. From the consultee's standpoint, consultation provides him with a professional resource which can aid him in performing his work-role without requiring him to obtain the training or to assume the role of the mental health professional.

Since mental health professionals are usually in the business of evaluating and treating disturbed people, it is understandable that the consultee may expect the consultant to see the consultee's clients. However, consultation does not involve the consultant dealing directly with the client for several reasons. In keeping with the goals mentioned above, the consultant helps the consultee deal with the client more effectively within the consultee-client relationship.

An essential element of consultation is familiarization of the consultant with the organization and functioning of the consultee system. Observation and understanding of police work-role activities is a necessary preliminary step toward effective consultation. Within this framework, the psychological consultants would be physically present in the police department regularly to consult with individual policemen regarding problem cases which they encountered in their work. This arrangement maximizes accessibility of the consultant and attempts to make contact with the consultant an integral part of the policemen's work shift.

In addition to this form of help, psychological consultants can perform other services which can improve the mental health functions of policemen. In designing this project, it was planned that these other activities could enhance the familiarization process for the consultants as well as provide needed services.

Training

In addition to the consultation activities just described, it was anticipated that the consultants could provide more formal training programs for groups of police officers, such as recruits, command and supervisory personnel, and other special groups. Possible training topics proposed were mental health problems, human relations, crisis intervention, interviewing and supervisory techniques.

Community Agency Cooperation

Discussions with police officials highlighted the limited resources they have for dealing with disturbed behavior beyond the initial stages of a crisis situation. They expressed their conviction that the physical environment of the police department and jail were inappropriate places for treating disturbed people, and they felt a great need for improved awareness on their part of referral sources, and for increased cooperation with other helping agencies.

Consultants can take a significant role in promoting cooperation between police and other community agencies in dealing with mental health problems. The consultants can maintain relationships with other agencies and provide a cross-agency perspective in the handling of multi-agency problems. One model which has proven effective in this regard is a continuous conference of workers from various agencies who meet regularly to discuss mutual problems, review cases in which several agencies are involved, and develop procedures for improving work with multi-agency problems (Rhodes, *et al.*, 1968).

In the particular case of Austin, it seemed that likely candidates for participants would be representatives of the various mental health facilities, family service, public health and welfare agencies, the schools, juvenile court, Council on Alcoholism and the Human Opportunities Corporation.[1] This activity would be coordinated with agencies which have broad program concerns, such as the Community Council, Austin-Travis County Mental Health Association, and the Community Mental Health-Mental Retardation Center. The goal of this conference was to increase the knowledge of the participants about the services and policies of each agency, and to facilitate interagency cooperation by promoting greater familiarity among the agency personnel. It was felt that more personal acquaintance among these workers would increase their readiness to communicate with each other regard-

---

[1] The Community Action Agency of the Office of Economic Opportunity.

ing mutual problems, which could in turn lead to more cooperation and better client services.

PROCEDURES

The project was conceived as a demonstration of this method of training, with the expectation that, if successful, the project would be continued by the City of Austin or some other source providing funds. The demonstration project ran from mid-November, 1969, through August, 1971.

The consultant staff was composed of a supervising consultant and advanced graduate students from the Community Mental Health Training Program, Department of Psychology, at the University of Texas. The student-consultants had received previous training and experience in clinical psychology and community mental health, and were receiving training in mental health consultation during the project.

The student-consultants spent a considerable portion of their initial work in the police department observing police procedures and familiarizing themselves with various aspects of police work. They accompanied police officers in their rounds, interviewed policemen concerning the operation of the department, and studied police records and documents to acquaint themselves with the kind and extent of police work with various problems.

EVALUATION

The effectiveness of a project such as this is admittedly difficult to assess, as it is with all such endeavors. Nevertheless, some attempt at evaluation is essential. The complexity of the problems addressed and the multiple goals pursued required the assessment of several different dimensions.

It is not feasible to reduce all of these dimensions to quantifiable attributes, nor even to obtain adequate data in relation to all of them. Additionally, the complicated set of social forces which may effect any given index makes interpretation of that data which is available quite difficult. This project was not conceived as an experimental intervention in the laboratory sense of the term, and police control groups were not included in the design, so that before and after comparisons of police behavior as reflected in police records are subject to many influences other than the consultation project.

Furthermore, there has been insufficient study of innovative programs of this type to provide a framework for establishing expectations. For some goals, the length of the project is probably sufficient to assess the effects of the project intervention; for others, a longer time period may be required and effects can only be assessed by subsequent evaluations. Finally, the project may fail to demonstrate changes anticipated in its design, but may result in unanticipated effects, both desirable and undesirable. Through searching review and analysis of procedures, every effort has been made to minimize undesirable effects, but one can hardly plan deliberately for unexpected benefits.

There are two types of evaluation relevant to projects such as this one. Caplan (1968) refers to these as evaluation of achievement and evaluation of process. Schulberg, Sheldon and Baker (1969) speak of goal-attainment models and systems models of evaluative research. While full discussion of these concepts is beyond the scope of this report, some elucidation of their main characteristics may be helpful. Evaluation of achievement is probably the most common approach to evaluation and simply involves setting some goals and assessing whether or not they are attained. Taking such an approach, the researcher assumes that the necessary resources to reach the goals will be allocated to the project, that critical sub- or intermediate goals will be attained, and that this will be reflected in the evaluation of outcome. The process or systems approach does not make these assumptions, but attempts to measure the allocation of resources and the attainment of subgoals as the program progresses. To employ this latter approach, one must be able to specify subgoals and to measure the various parameters involved, which admittedly is a more complicated and expensive procedure. However, one accrues the advantage of being able to provide feedback and hopefully to effect program modifications as processes are seen not to articulate with subgoals within the conduct of the program. This approach allows the generation of more knowledge about the phenomena under study and is particularly applicable to situations where information about program expectations and the effectiveness of various interventions is limited. Perhaps more importantly, the analysis of process and system should provide greater generalizability to other situations which may differ in one or more respects from the demonstration situation. A third type of evaluation, called administrative evaluation by Caplan, and evaluation of efficiency by Schulberg, Sheldon and Baker, would seem necessarily to come after the process and achievement types of evaluation in most instances, although the systems approach does provide for some attention to this type of assessment. However, evaluation of efficiency is generally beyond the scope of this project, and it will be possible only to make some general comments about efficiency from the review of other types of evaluative data.

Within the limitations of time allotted to this project and the uncertainty of the expectations which might be set for it, it seemed most sound to proceed within a process model of evaluation. While the ultimate goal of this program would require some measurement of the mental health of the community, assessment of such a goal far exceeds the ambitions of this project. Effecting the mental health of a community by the indirect means of diffusion of knowledge through several intermediaries requires careful assessment of the intermediate goals. Thus, in general, research on mental health consultation has to date been limited largely to the assessment of its effects on consultees (Mannino and Shore, 1971). It is apparent that the many difficulties in achieving these effects will need to be ironed out before meaningful effects on entire populations can be assessed.

Accordingly, this report is devoted primarily to a careful description of what was done, what resources were allocated, what obstacles were encountered, and what has been learned from the experience that might improve such efforts in the future. Survival of the program, in the form of its continuation beyond the funded period may well be the most meaningful criterion for this project. However, some data on the achievement of intermediate goals can be presented which are based on the social-psychological theories underlying this type of intervention.

One set of data is based on analysis of police reports of interventions in family disturbances. Samples of these reports were collected for randomly selected periods at the beginning and end of the project. The nature of the intervention, as best it could be assessed from the reports, was compared for these two time periods. Since these reports are typically not considered highly important in police work and records are frequently sketchy if completed at all (Bard, 1970), these data will be limited to assessing types of interventions, rather than effectiveness.

A second set of data involved analysis of the proportion of referrals to the Community Mental Health-Mental Retardation Center from police sources at the beginning and end of the project. Since increasing policemen's awareness of referral sources was one of the intermediate goals of the project, the number of such referrals was expected to increase.

A third set of data is composed of attitude questionnaires administered to members of the police department at the beginning and end of the project. A seventy-two-item questionnaire dealing with the handling of the mentally disturbed in the community was constructed (See Appendix II) by the consultants based on what they had discovered through their familiarization activities to be salient issues for the police in the field of mental health. This scale and Fessler's (1952) *C-Scale,* which is designed to measure cohesiveness of community attitudes, were administered to all commissioned members of the police department, and to staff members of the Community Mental Health-Mental Retardation Center and the Austin State Hospital on a before and after basis. It was expected that the scores of the policemen and the mental health workers should show increasing convergence over time as an index of the achievement of greater contact and familiarity among them through the efforts of the consultants.

Inasmuch as this project was designed as a cooperative training endeavor, it is also important to assess the impact of the program on the students who participated as consultants and on the contribution this experience has made to their professional training. This will necessarily be done anecdotally, based on changes in their attitudes and behavior expressed in supervisory sessions as well as their behavior as consultants.

More broadly, it is hoped that the report of this project can contribute to the body of knowledge which psychologists and other social scientists require to improve their efforts to achieve greater cooperation and integration of the major institutions of American society (Bard, 1969B). In another sense, then, reports such as this one constitute process evaluations within the larger enterprise of community psychology, a relatively new field in the behavioral sciences seeking to help communities with the process of change.

Chapter II

FAMILIARIZATION AND ITS LESSONS

THE DEFINITION OF PROBLEMS

EFFORTS TO FAMILIARIZE the consultants with police work began with the selection of two advanced graduate students to work on the project during the first year. Reading materials were assigned, discussion of consultation techniques were held, and visits to the police department were made.

Familiarization is a critical phase in the consultation process (Mann, 1971). The initial orientation visits were intended to provide knowledge of the department's organizational structure, to gain an understanding of the roles and responsibilities of various personnel, as well as to meet them personally, and to begin to promote some visibility for the consultation project. The consultant's orientation at this point is to act as if he were a student of the policemen, in order to acquire knowledge about normal and routine police operations, as well as problem areas, so that later consultative interventions will be consonant with the policeman's operational patterns.

In order to facilitate the familiarization process, we joined the Police Buddy Program, an existing activity in which citizens may sign up to ride with police officers. This experience provided an impression of what it feels like to be *processed,* including fingerprinting, mug shots, completing forms, and having a police records check completed. All police buddies are given name tags indicating their status; a concession was made for our tags to read *Police Consultant.*

While this process served to ease us into an existing program of access to riding with policemen, it created some problems of confused identity. On the one hand there were those in the department who were disenchanted with the Police Buddy Program, but there were other groups, such as law students, participating in the Police Buddy Program for other reasons. These factors tended to obscure both our identity and purposes and to influence the nature of the entry problem.

Ordinarily the entry of consultants into a client-system creates some imbalance of organizational structure, and while this poses a problem with which the consultant must deal, it also heightens his visibility, and provides some leverage for establishing relationships within the organization. The fact that we could fit into an existing program in the system made physical and logistical entry easier, but created other problems of psychological entry.

Since the organizational structure of the department offered no alternative, this problem was accepted as one of the obstacles to be overcome in working with this particular social system. Nevertheless, the problem of visibility was to command our continuing attention.

The visibility problem was particularly strong for the student consultants, who were initially less well known in the department than was the supervising consultant. Again, this situation produced an interesting variation from the expectations of consultation theory. While the age and appearance of the student consultants led them to be easily confused with other students in the Police Buddy Program, these same features made it easier for them to establish relationships with some of the younger patrolmen than was true for the supervising consultant.

Caplan (1970) suggests that the consultant should strive to establish a coordinate relationship with the consultee in order to minimize problems which may arise from consultant-consultee status differences. One would expect that the student consultants could accomplish this aspect of the relationship easily with younger patrolmen, an expectation which proved to be correct. However, because of the hierarchical nature of the police organization, coordinate relationships of this sort create other problems. In this project, at least, it was difficult for the student consultants to maintain roles as both coordinate workers and change agents, since their interventions could be neutralized quickly by supervisory personnel with whom the student consultants had not established similar relationships. Since contact between supervisors and consultants was less than optimal because of the logistical arrangements of the project, this also remained a persistent obstacle, and more discussion of this issue will be presented in a later chapter.

Another administrative decision was to assign the responsibility for the program within the department to the Police-Community Relations Officer. This, too, had to be viewed as a mixed blessing. The Police-Community Relations Officer was at a disadvantage in that he had not participated in the planning of the project and was unfamiliar with its objectives. Moreover, he was overworked already with little assistance for carrying out extensive responsibilities.[2] Assignment of the project to him proved to be part of an established routine of shuttling many such special projects to the Community Relations Office.

We were aware that police-community relations functions are viewed at best as auxiliary activities, and at worst as communist-inspired foreign incursions, in many police departments. Therefore, it seemed imperative that the project achieve a degree of autonomy and that we relate actively to the several elements of the department.

The Police-Community Relations Officer was not unaware of these problems, and proved to be extremely helpful in introducing us to various key members of the department, in anticipating problems and in taking the time from his overcrowded schedule to discuss problems and provide *inside* assistance. It happened that this particular officer had excellent personal relationships throughout the department, which were established through his long experience on the force. Consequently, the project benefitted, on the whole, from its association with the community relations function. Under other conditions, such an arrangement might not have been desirable.

The Austin Police Department is organized into three primary

---

[2] As of this writing, the Police-Community Relations office has been expanded in staff, resources and facilities as the result of a grant awarded to the department. We were able to play a role in the development of this program, participate as resource people in several community-relations activities, and to help in designing training sessions in community relations. Although this was not a feature of the original conception of the project, this outcome illustrates one of the unanticipated benefits referred to earlier.

elements: The Uniformed Division, which is primarily responsible for patrol functions; the Criminal Investigation Division, which specializes in investigative work, and the Service Division, which handles mainly training responsibilities. Various activities required coordination with all three of these divisions. For example, it was necessary to confer with the chain of command in the Service Division to organize a training activity and to coordinate with the command of one or both of the other divisions to schedule personnel to attend the training.

Similarly, while most of the crisis-oriented work with disturbed and/or disturbing persons is done by the Uniform Division, primary responsibility for such cases is assigned to the Homicide Detail of the Criminal Investigation Division.[3] Thus, there are built-in organizational problems in coordinating the efforts of the department as a whole around the question of dealing with disturbed people.

One might say that with respect to behavior falling within the purview of the police there is *first-line* responsibility and there is *real* responsibility. Thus, for example, patrol personnel are responsible for responding to initial reports of burglary. If they have a *hot* report, they may apprehend a suspect and exercise primary responsibility. But in the majority of cases, the patrol officer takes a report from a complainant hours or even days after the burglary occurs and refers the report to the Burglary Detail of the Criminal Investigation Division, which then assumes responsibility for solving the case. The patrolman's main activities in handling such a case are making an arrest and filing a report.

In dealing with disturbed people, the patrolman tends to be influenced toward following an analogous procedure. That is, if

---

[3] At first glance, this arrangement seems to reflect an antiquated attitude that the mentally ill are homicidal or suicidal, and perhaps historically this is true. However, the major reason for this division of labor seems to be that, under the law, policemen can intervene officially with disturbed people only when those people are dangerous to themselves or others. This arrangement ignores the far more numerous situations of family disturbances which are not specifically covered by law and where the policeman's power to intervene officially is quite limited. This organizational arrangement would seem to perpetuate any existing attitude that the mentally ill are dangerous but those Homicide Detail personnel who had close contact with disturbed persons did not seem to hold such attitudes.

he cannot make an arrest, there is a tendency to refer the case to the Criminal Investigation Division which is viewed as having *real* responsibility for such cases. In the case of a family disturbance report, unless there is some violation of law to which the patrolman is witness, no legal action can be taken without a formal complaint. Patrolmen are instructed to tell the complaining party to file a written complaint at the police station under such circumstances, and typically take no further action. Since most complainants do not wish to file formal charges, including many who initially say that they will do so and then later change their minds after the passions of the moment have subsided, the possibility for further intervention is usually aborted at this point. Policemen are aware that family disturbances are potentially dangerous situations, and they are instructed to limit their interventions and leave the scene as quickly as possible. The Homicide Detail cannot be called into such situations under the circumstances, and the result is that the combination of legal and organizational assignments of responsibility leave no one to assume responsibility for further intervention. Tacit recognition of this state of affairs is reflected in relatively inadequate reports and record keeping in this area even though it comprises a large proportion of police business.

One could enter a philosophical discourse at this point about the questions of individual and social responsibility, the burden of initiating help-seeking, etc. The fact remains that the individuals involved in a family disturbance have asked for help. From the perspective of an informed outsider, it is possible to say that they have sought the wrong kind of help, and clinical practitioners of mental health might question their motivations. However, these judgements assume an awareness of community resources which does not exist in reality among the general population and overlook the fact that many people see the police as a logical help-giving resource (Liberman, 1969). Thus, the question becomes one of the patrolman responding to the request for help in ways which are appropriate to the request and within his legally and organizationally defined functions.

The familiarization experience revealed that few of the policemen knew of community referral sources for mental health problems, that the existence and location of the community mental health center was not well known, and that the policeman who had been inside the county unit of the state mental hospital was rare indeed.

As familiarization progressed, the fact that the supervising consultant received several telephone requests for help from persons who had been advised to call by policemen was further evidence of the lack of knowledge of, or lack of faith in, community resources. At the same time, these calls testified to the patrolmen's willingness to use referral sources about which they had knowledge.

Several officers mentioned their need for such information when questioned about it, emphasizing that if the information were in convenient form, such as a shirt-pocket sized card, it would be more likely to be used. All officers had been given directories of community services previously, but these were usually misplaced or discarded because they were inconvenient to carry. In addition to suggesting that specific referral information in usuable form was needed, this information also indicated that the planned series of meetings between community agency representatives and policemen could be quite helpful.

A significant part of the familiarization experiences consisted of riding with policemen on patrol. Logs were kept of these experiences, which formed an important data base for planning activities in the project during supervisory sessions. From our standpoint as consultants, the modal character of these experiences for policemen seemed to be dullness and routine. For the seasoned policemen, the typical activity of a patrol is singularly unexciting: taking reports of thefts which may have occurred several days ago; maintaining a visible presence; and filling out numerous forms. Since the intended purpose of patrol duty is to provide a deterrent effect, this is as it should be. However, those events which are unusual or dangerous seem all the more emotionally arousing by contrast. At this latter end of the spectrum, we had the experience of accompanying officers in answering family disturbance calls which verged on violence, and in making routine arrests for misdemeanor offenses in which smouldering racial tensions threatened to explode into physical combat. Although instances of actual violence in situations of both these types occurred during the course of the project, no such instances occurred when we were present.

Among those events which we did witness, it would be difficult to critize the actions of the policemen when all of the factors in the situation are taken into account. Most often, we were left with the conclusion that things could best be improved if the situation were different prior to the occurrence of the incident. Although there were instances in which different police behavior would have had more desirable effect on that particular situation, there were usually other considerations which made it seem that, under the circumstances, teaching policemen techniques to handle such situations would not alter the situation as much as would changing the definition of the situation in the eyes of both the police and the public. Thus, preventive efforts related to police-citizen interaction might well focus on attempts to change the way the participants define the situation.

We witnessed numerous incidents of police intervention which were handled effectively. The major differentiating factor in effective and ineffective handling of human conflict situations seemed to be the priorities which operated in a given event. To exemplify this point, a hypothetical event will be described, which is composed of elements of several actual incidents arranged so as to protect the confidentiality of the participants.

While on a night stake-out for drug abuse suspects, a uniformed patrolman is approached by a woman from a nearby ethnic minority neighborhood who identifies a boy passing by as having committed several misdemeanor thefts in the area. The patrolman follows the boy home to investigate further, accompanied by the woman. The woman identifies some things in the boy's yard as stolen items. As the patrolman begins to question the boy, the boy's father comes out of the house to join the discussion. The father demands to know why the boy is being questioned and at the same instant the boy starts to walk into the house. In short order, the policeman places the boy under arrest, the father tries to intervene and is also arrested, and an angry mob of neighborhood residents gathers and begins to shout at the policeman. As tempers mount and a violent confrontation appears imminent, the policeman warns the crowd back, forces the boy and the father into the patrol car and leaves the scene quickly, while the crowd believes they have witnessed another scene of police harassment.

Subsequent investigation revealed that the boy had a history of minor juvenile offenses, poor school adjustment and was considered mildly mentally retarded. The father, who was dressed in faded work clothes at the time of the incident, was a responsible businessman. He objected strenuously to what he thought was precipitous action by the policeman. This scene is repeated frequently in one form or another in most urban areas, and because of its potential for creating community unrest and public violence deserves further analysis.

The policeman explained his actions as follows. He knew of a large number of reported thefts in the area, and such cases are quite difficult to solve. He felt that he had enough evidence to warrant further investigation, but the boy's entry into the house would have thwarted his efforts, since he could not obtain a warrant for his arrest on a misdemeanor charge. Thus, he felt obliged to make an arrest. He was in an ethnic minority neighborhood where he was unfamiliar with either the locale or the residents. As the crowd gathered, he was aware of potential danger, and felt the best solution was to clear out before the situation became worse. He interpreted the actions of the father and the crowd as resistance and felt that forceful action was necessary to hasten his departure.

Persons in the crowd were interviewed subsequently. In their view, the crowd saw a policeman forcibly arresting a boy and a man. The residents of the neighborhood, which has a relatively low crime rate, higher than average percentage of homeowners, and higher socioeconomic status residents than most comparable neighborhoods of similar ethnic composition in the community, wanted an explanation for this incident which seemed unjustified in view of their law-abiding image of themselves. When they did not receive one, they felt the surge of discrimination and oppression which has been part of their cultural experience. The incident clearly left a bad taste in their mouths, and while a full-scale riot seems unlikely to occur in this neighborhood, the residents' image of the police acquired an additional increment of tarnish.

One cannot evaluate such an event without being sympathetic to both points of view. The policeman acted successfully from a crime-apprehension standpoint and avoided what he thought was potential physical threat to himself. Under similar circumstances, it is not inconceivable that other officers might have drawn firearms, and having done so, might have had to use them. The crowd acted understandably from a territorial protection perspective, and seeing the policeman as an outsider, felt entitled to an explanation of the intervention.

The critical issues this event raises for the creation of more effective community life are complex indeed. There are conflicts between short and long-term goals, and between law-enforcement and order-maintenance priorities which none of the participants can be expected to resolve adequately during the incident itself. No one can deny the policeman's right to make an arrest and to protect himself; yet, no one can deny the fairness of the residents' desire for an explanation. Thus, successful conduct of the law-enforcement function may have diminished respect for authority generally in the neighborhood, thus making order maintenance, and perhaps subsequent law enforcement, more difficult.[4]

One could not advocate logically that nonenforcement of the law would be a successful solution. It might have reduced the immediate angry reaction of the crowd, but could have the same long-range effect of decreasing respect for the law. It seems unlikely that the policeman could have made a successful explanation of the complicated reasons for his actions to the onlookers given his assessment of the potential for violence in the situation. Therefore, information and understanding must predate such events. At best, only partial improvement can result from looking at the incident itself and such solutions are likely to conflict with other goals.

Had the policeman and the residents been more familiar with each other there could have been much less of a sense of urgency on both sides, which seems to have been the major disruptive

---

[4] Police action is more likely to draw a crowd in minority neighborhoods than other neighborhoods according to Bittner (1970).

force in this situation. Such knowledge would have to come from police-community interaction prior to the event, and would have to be in the form of a behavioral setting which did not involve law enforcement since the latter tends to bias the samples of both policemen and citizens.

One cannot expect the residents to know the technicalities of the law, but the community does expect the policeman to have such knowledge. If specialized knowledge is a hallmark of a profession, then it is reasonable to expect the members of a profession to have all the knowledge that is necessary to do their job. In this case, specialized sociological knowledge of the neighborhood and a more accurate picture of the neighborhood crime statistics would have been helpful, but it is becoming increasingly clear that one of the prerequisites for effective police functioning is to know about and to be known by the various members of the community on a personal basis.

On an anecdotal level, the effects of familiarity can be seen in changes in the attitudes of the student consultants as they became familiar with the policeman's role. Initially, some of their attitudes toward the police were similar to the stereotypes held by many people. Their views of policemen ranged from seeing them as strongly authoritarian and aggressive to assuming that they were unsophisticated and dull. While the greatest changes usually accompanied their first patrol ride, there was a gradual increase in appreciation of the reasons for police behavior, recognition of the effective work they do under difficult conditions and awareness of the community pressures they face. The students discovered the thorough training which the policemen receive, the number of policemen with college training in psychology, sociology, and law, and the common sense attitudes about behavior which the policemen bring to their job.

Without exception, these lessons helped to make the student consultants' attitudes toward the police more positive, and their orientation to *change-agentry* both more realistic and more challenging. As consultants, the students were able to face problem situations with a greater sharing of goals and perceptions with policemen, realizing that needed changes were sometimes beyond the officer-subject interaction.

Perhaps as a result of this process of familiarization and improved understanding, we began to consider increasingly the effects of exposure to selected samples of community life on the attitudes of the policemen as well. One of these factors is the socioeconomic background from which policemen are recruited (Lipset, 1969). Illustrative of this point is the remark one policeman made in evaluating a course in psychology which was taught for members of the department. Asked how the course had changed him, the officer replied that he now felt more confident in dealing with persons who were better educated than he was (Mann, 1970). More broadly, this background limits the diversity of social experiences, norms and attitudes in the community with which the policeman is familiar. The selectivity of the policeman's prior experience is evidenced by Sterling and Watson's (1970) finding that police recruits have had strikingly low geographical mobility in an era in which geographical mobility in the general population is increasing dramatically.

A second obvious selective factor is the bias in the subsamples of various population groups with which the policeman is likely to have official contact. A few examples should illustrate this point dramatically: the homicidal and suicidal among the mentally disturbed; the senile and confused among the aged; the neglected, deprived poor delinquent and the neglected, overindulged affluent delinquent among the young; and the criminal and socially irresponsible subsample of the population in general. Social class and cultural factors also introduce systematic biases into the visibility and definition of deviant behavior (Gans, 1962; Rhodes, in press). The resulting combination of selective stimulus characteristics to which the policeman is exposed make it difficult to imagine how the policeman might avoid constructing stereotypes which are more or less true to his experience, unless he has training to improve his assessment of human behavior in such settings.

We were impressed with the techniques which the policemen had developed for handling a variety of difficult situations with which most people, including behavioral scientists, are rarely confronted. The time and intensity pressures under which most of these techniques are employed lead to such techniques becoming routine procedures, often nearly reflexive reactions. This state of affairs increases the sense of security and confidence with which the officer operates under otherwise trying conditions, but it would also seem to make the patterns of practice extremely refractive to change on the basis of routine experience alone. Often there is little opportunity for reflection about the relationship between the assumptions an officer makes and the particular technique he employs in a given situation. Compared to knowledge of the law and departmental policies covering other situations, much less time and importance is given to learning to assess the social psychological situation and to developing psychological techniques of intervention. Yet it is the application of the stereotype to cases which do not fit it that makes the use of techniques based on such assessments ineffective, that creates concern among policemen and other citizens about the proper handling of disturbed behavior, and which may frustrate even the policeman who is committed to helping people to the extent that he may lapse into self-fulfilling, pessimistic assumptions about his own efficacy in such cases. These impressions need to be integrated into a theoretical framework for intervention, which is the subject of the next chapter.

In summary, the familiarization phase of the project helped to teach us about the policeman's role, routine, and organizational relationships in ways which helped to define problems, and illuminated avenues and barriers to be observed in seeking the solutions. At the same time, the complexities and subtleties involved in the relationship between a community and one of its major institutions are so numerous that these observations and proposed solutions must be regarded as tentative and subject to re-evaluation and revision. In a real sense, the familiarization process is unending, and at no time did we have the feeling that we had run its full course.

Chapter III

THEORETICAL BACKGROUND

Nothing is so practical as a good theory.
—Kurt Lewin

THERE IS NO COMPREHENSIVE theory which could guide intervention into the complex community processes surrounding a major social institution and its clients. We had to rely on a multiplicity of theoretical ideas drawn from several disciplines, and to test and modify these notions at the same time that we used them as tentative guidelines. The assumptions of sociology and demography as they relate to mental illness have been mentioned in Chapter I, and organizational theories can help in understanding some of the dynamics of the police organization itself. However, we also needed an action theory of change which could guide our efforts within the sociological and organizational frameworks outlining some dimensions of the problem. It is this latter aspect which is the contribution of community psychology.

As clinical psychologists, we were familiar with theories of therapeutic change, some of which have been extended to apply to group techniques and to consultation methods which are not explicitly therapeutic. While these concepts provided an important basis for our understanding of human behavior and its change, there is also a body of theory dealing with attitude formation and change which we felt would be helpful since it was not developed from theories of abnormal personality and does not require any assumptions about pathology. This is an important consideration, since psychological consultants have to be prepared to deal with the expectations of consultees which stem from the widespread tendency to see psychologists as *shrinks*. Experienced consultants have had to learn to avoid the trap of yielding to the occasional subtle invitation to assume the role of therapist, a pressure which was also encountered in this project. Therefore, we tried to rely as much as possible on theoretical ideas which were not rooted in pathology, and on techniques which did not have a distinctly psychotherapeutic tinge.

Another important limitation on the utility of therapeutically oriented theory and technique involved the logistics of the project. We could not expect to have a significant impact on an organization of over 300 personnel through individual, one-to-one interventions with front-line workers simply because of the time limitations involved. In addition, any gains which might be made with individuals in this way would have to be regarded as fragile and subject to change from any counteracting organizational or situational forces.

Finally, we had to recognize that the ultimate targets of our efforts at intervention were not the policemen themselves but people in the community, most often disturbed people. We saw the policeman as facing an exacting task of trying to influence people in situations characterized by personal and interpersonal strain of various types, in which the policeman's usual reliance on force and authority would be frequently inappropriate. From a psychological standpoint, influence attempts of this kind require the policeman to be able to *get close* to the people and to try to assess and understand the situational pressures the people were experiencing. These considerations indicated that we would have to try to influence the policeman's attitude toward disturbed behavior as well as to teach knowledge and skills for handling disturbed people, and we needed to define a theoretical basis for attitude change and training.

Encounter Groups and Sensitivity Training

A frequent response to perceived needs for changing policemen's attitudes (a need sometimes not shared by the policemen involved) in recent years has been to initiate programs of police-community interaction under controlled circumstances, either through varieties of confrontation, sensitivity, or encounter groups (Sikes and Cleveland, 1968; Lipsitt and Steinbruner, 1969) or programs such as the Police Buddy Plan described earlier. While there is evidence that the intergroup contacts which these programs provide are a necessary element in promoting greater familiarity between policemen and other community members, it cannot be assumed that changes in individual attitudes subsequent to such contacts are sufficient to foster improved conditions in the community. Evaluations of these group projects do show changes in attitudes, but the attitudes of community members show more change than do those of the policemen, and the changes in police attitudes are frequently short-lived when tested on follow-ups (Sacon, 1971). Moreover, the relationship between attitudes and behavior is not a simple one, and is highly dependent on situational factors which exist in the natural environment, as distinct from the artificial setting of the encounter group (Fried, 1968). Evaluation of such programs requires both attitudinal and behavioral measures. Programs such as the Buddy Plan have not been systematically evaluated, but one would expect that they would mainly change the attitudes of the Buddies, since they are conducted on the policeman's turf and tend to have an unrepresentative sample of community participants.

Both of these approaches tend to ignore organizational and work-role sources of attitude maintenance which impose strong forces against lasting attitude change on the part of policemen as a result of short-term interventions. The social psychological dynamics of these forces and recommendations for dealing with the problem of police-community familiarity more generally are discussed in detail in subsequent chapters of this report.

A final limitation on the encounter group approach is that they do not lend themselves to teaching the knowledge and skills which it was assumed were necessary in this project. Accordingly, group sessions of this type were not considered a sufficient means for accomplishing the goals of the program.

Already, the reader will begin to appreciate the complexity of the problem, and the reasons for the fact that this document will not satisfy those who would like to see some results based on systematic testing of hypotheses. As theorists, we had to be very pragmatic, but we felt that theory could provide an important roadmap as long as we didn't use it slavishly in those instances where it didn't match the terrain we encountered.

In general, we relied on three kinds of theories: consultation theory, theories of attitude change, and theories of group dynamic approaches to organizational behavior. In this chapter, our expectations based on these theories will be discussed. Later, the limitations and needed modifications of these concepts, as well as the needs for other theories which the project suggests, can be examined in the light of our actual experience.

Mental Health Consultation Theory

Gerald Caplan has developed a theory of mental health consultation based on a model of consultees voluntarily seeking out a mental health professional for help with a specific work-related problem (1970). While Caplan discusses several types of consultation, consideration will be given here to the type of consultation in which specific changes are sought in the consultee, since this type of consultation is most germane to the project under discussion. Caplan refers to this type of consultation as consultee-centered. The rationale of a consultation approach, and its role in overall mental health strategies, have been discussed in Chapter I. It is important to bear in mind that this type of consultation rests on the consultee's initiative to bring problems to the consultant, and that consultation differs from psychotherapy in that it is limited to dealing with problems in the consultee's work role, not in his personality.

Caplan recognizes four types of activities in the consultee-centered approach to consultation, depending on the consultant's diagnosis of the problem which prompted the consultee to present the case to the consultant. These are a lack of knowledge, a lack of skill, a lack of confidence, or a lack of objectivity. However, he feels that each of the first three of these problems can be dealt with most effectively by referring back to the training or supervisory systems of the consultee's organization, or by the consultant working with groups of consultees. Caplan feels that the fourth type of problem must be handled on an individual basis and is not presently susceptible to group-based intervention. Since we were the training system for mental health problems in this project, we had to assume the responsibility for working with the policemen on problems of knowledge, skill and confidence, but

Caplan's theory of consultation seems to offer little help in these areas. Before discussing training strategies, however, it will be helpful to consider Caplan's ideas on the problem of objectivity, since this condition may exist with or without adequate knowledge and skill.

Examination of Caplan's notions about objectivity problems in consultees reveals why he does not feel group methods are appropriate. He proposes that consultees may be hampered in dealing with certain types of clients because their problems are similar to some conflict-laden experience in the consultee's own background. Rather than seeing the problem objectively, the consultee's perception of the problem is distorted by the *theme* surrounding his own experience with a similar problem. This *theme interference* then becomes the focus of the consultant's change efforts.

According to Caplan, themes take the form of a syllogism. If the consultee perceives the client as fitting a certain *initial category,* for instance, *coming from a broken home,* then the consultee will assume that the client will suffer an *inevitable outcome* linked by the theme to the *initial category,* for example, *leading a life of crime.* Both the *initial category* and the *inevitable outcome* are assumed to be associated with the consultee's own history of conflict. Since the consultant does not explore the consultee's own history or dynamics, as might be done in psychotherapy, it is possible to intervene in such themes by showing the consultee that either the client does not fit the *initial category,* or that the *outcome* is not inevitable. Caplan prefers the latter approach, since he believes that the former only establishes the client as an exception to categorization and does not reduce the consultee's theme. Caplan claims that demonstrating the fallacy of the *inevitable outcome* assumption through careful examination of the client's behavior does reduce theme interference, and he presents some evidence to support his contention (1970, Chapt. 12). Since themes are idiosyncratic, they cannot be reduced by applying this technique to groups of consultees.

Caplan's model for theme interference and his technique for reducing it would fit many types of stereotyped thinking and prejudiced attitudes. We anticipated that the theme interference hypothesis would be a good prototype for analyzing problems of objectivity. However, it is not always necessary to invoke the dynamics of intrapsychic conflict to explain such phenomena, since stereotyped attitudes leading to syllogistic oversimplifications can be held on the basis of incorrect information and maintained by superficial and limited exposure to contradictory facts. To the extent that such beliefs are shared by members of a group and associated with group norms regarding behavior, they may acquire as much, if not more, of the strength and emotional connotations which Caplan attributes to intrapsychic dynamics.

Since Caplan's techniques of consultation rest on the consultee's conflict producing motivation for change, it is not clear that the same type of intervention techniques would apply equally to all such instances of stereotyping. Further, the fact that the technique relies on one-to-one transactions means that it would not produce as widespread an effect as we were hoping to accomplish in this project, and would not fit with many of the larger scale intervention strategies which we planned to employ. Thus, while we planned to employ case consultation methods we did not consider these alone to be sufficient for accomplishing our goals.

Attitudes and Attitude Change[5]

Since we were prepared to help policemen with problems of knowledge and skill in group training sessions, it was desirable that we include in these sessions some techniques for dealing with objectivity. We assumed that a central stereotype which we would have to change was the widespread belief that the mentally ill are

---

[5] A special acknowledgement is due the work of Morton Bard (1970), whose work in training teams of police specialists to work with family crises in New York has been helpful in planning this project. Many of our ideas have been stimulated by his reports and by personal communications. An important difference between his project and this one is that the geographical concentration of the police precinct in which he worked made the use of a specialist team approach workable, whereas the geographical dispersion of the city of Austin made such an approach impractical. Family crisis teams would not be able to respond quickly enough to situations scattered potentially from one end of the city to the other. Thus, we had to develop a generalist approach, attempting to influence eventually the work of every officer on the force. This meant that we could not employ the intensive work with a small group of men which marked Bard's work, and also that we had less control over reporting and record keeping procedures than was true in his project.

dangerous, and that many other attitudes and practices would be linked to this belief. This assumption was based on the fact that the attitudinal linkage between mental illness and dangerousness has broad popular and historical support in our culture, and the high probability that many of the policemen were likely to remember more vividly incidents which reinforced this connection than those which disconfirmed the belief. We further assumed that this belief would be reinforced in police cadet training, not only because of the attitudes of senior policemen, but also because the policemen's legal basis for intervening with disturbed people is based primarily on their contention that the latter are dangerous to themselves or others. Using these assumptions, it was not necessary to make inferences about the presence of psychological conflicts in order to define a problem with which we could work.

Observations of police training indicated that attitudes were not taught directly, but rather were induced indirectly from teaching techniques and skills. For instance, police cadets were exposed to a practical problem situation in which a beserk man was firing a gun wildly from inside a building. The problem was acted out with considerable realism, including the firing of blank ammunition. A squad of cadets was assigned to handle the situation without specific instructions. Since many of the cadets were military veterans, this problem was typically handled as one might expect to see an army squad surround and capture or kill an enemy sniper. There are important tactical lessons to be learned from such experiences, and certainly policemen must be prepared to deal with such situations whether they involve someone who is disturbed or an individual who has committed a crime and is attempting to avoid capture. The object of this particular lesson, however, was supposed to be to alert the cadets to the fact that the subject was not firing *at* anyone in particular and that their first response should not be to kill the man, but rather to try to apprehend him. Needless to say, this subtle distinction was lost on many cadets until after the exercise was over. Aside from learning techniques, however, this exercise seemed highly likely to induce, or at least support, the attitude that mentally ill persons are dangerous. The theme of emphasizing the dangerous aspects of several practical police situations ran through much of the training experiences of the cadets.[6]

Alerting the police cadet to potentially dangerous situations is, of course, an important and indispensable part of his training. It would be misleading to merely attempt to teach him a general attitude that the mentally ill are not dangerous, since this might conflict with his other training. At the same time, it seemed important to counteract the attitude that mental illness and dangerousness were highly correlated, and to present the cadets with a wider range of disturbed behavior so that they could learn to distinguish people more accurately according to the potential danger they posed. In situations such as the one described above, the policeman's prior attitude about mental illness and danger would strongly influence his perception of the situation.

Our analysis of the problem seemed to fit well with the findings of research on attitudes that exposure to new stimuli tends to enhance the attractiveness of the stimuli (Zajonc, 1968) and from research on interpersonal attraction that proximity, and hence, increased exposure, increases the attractiveness of others (Berscheid and Walster, 1969). From a similar formulation in intergroup contact theory, it has been shown that increased contact between racial groups results in improved intergroup attitudes (Pettigrew, 1969).

We reasoned that similar effects could be expected from exposing policemen to new information about people exhibiting disturbed behavior and from actual exposure to persons with emotional problems in non-threatening situations. We also recognized that mere exposure would have to be accompanied by other activities which could enhance the probability of psychological exposure resulting from physical proximity and to tie the expected attitude changes to new techniques and skills.

---

[6] When asked about this phenomenon, senior police officers explained that their main goal in cadet training was to teach the potential officer to protect himself, and to recognize and handle dangerous situations. They assumed that he would learn more of the subtleties of handling such situations more positively through experience. However, we observed no deliberate effort to accomplish this latter goal through specific in-service training programs for experienced personnel. Most in-service training time was allocated to supervisory and leadership training, and specialized situational training occasioned by crises such as the rising frequency of protest demonstrations.

Training Strategies

From research on learning and attitude change, it is clear that both are enhanced when the subjects are active and involved in the process through which they are to receive new information. In order to emphasize this dimension, it was decided to employ training techniques which involved the policemen in role-playing practical problem situations whenever possible.

Because our analysis of the attitude problem assumed a commonly shared attitude tied to group norms, it was necessary to take account of group dynamics operating in both the training situation and subsequent experience. To use Lewin's (1951) terms, we attempted first to *unfreeze* the existing attitude, to change it, and then to *refreeze* the attitude on a new level. Doing so in a group setting should serve to change the group norm as it exposes all members of the group to new information, since the norm is assumed to develop out of a shared belief. Training sessions were planned to present initially some practical problem situations which would elicit the stereotyped response and disconfirm it, followed by a reassessment of the situation and instruction in techniques for handling it effectively. The final practical problem situations were presented so that the relationship between mental disturbance and expected behavior was ambiguous, and the problems required the trainee to make use of new information and skills in assessing and dealing with the situation. Group incentives were present in that each trainee role-played the problem situation in front of an audience of his fellow trainees.

We also considered the attitudes and practices of other groups in the community toward emotional disturbance, and the policemen's awareness of these phenomena. Police encounters with behavior in the community, including disturbed behavior, occur typically under conditions of relative social isolation, and the policemen's sense of loneliness in dealing with disturbed behavior was underscored by the lack of acquaintance with community referral sources, their frequent expressions of the wish that someone else in the community would help with such problems and, indeed, their request for consultative help from us. In turn, this condition indicates a relative isolation of the community agencies concerned with mental health from the police, and historically, from the community as a whole.

The absence of significant informational and attitudinal input from the mental health professional part of the community was seen as a problem which required more than the mere presence of consultants for its alleviation. On the one hand, closer contact and familiarity between mental health workers and policemen was considered necessary to achieve better coordination and more effective intervention into community mental health problems, and would help to further the community orientation which mental health agencies were beginning to develop at that time. On the other hand, to the extent that increased contact with mental health workers served to provide the policeman with more alternatives for dealing with disturbed people in an informational sense, and with the feeling that he was not as isolated in encountering disturbed behavior as he might have felt otherwise in an attitudinal sense, it was expected that these activities would bolster his confidence and reinforce the attitudinal and technical acquisitions resulting from training.

However, turning attention to other mental health agencies in the community brought to light another important issue in intergroup relations. At the time the project was getting under way there was a strong controversy between the state hospital and the police department resulting from a difference of opinion over the security measures taken with patients. The controversy was exacerbated by its becoming a political football involving not only the community, but also the state mental health system. While the majority of policemen were not directly involved, there was an antagonism between the two institutions at the administrative and supervisory levels which threatened to create disruption and poor cooperation in the handling of disturbed people, which could also counteract the attitudinal changes we were trying to accomplish through training.

This state of affairs increased the importance of the interagency meetings which were part of the original plan of the project. Using a theoretical approach similar to that proposed for the training sessions, we reasoned that bringing police administrators and supervisors together with mental health workers would provide exposure and contact which could lead to improved relationships between the personnel involved. By focusing these meetings on common problems, we hoped to make use of Sherif's (1958) concept of superordinate goals in reducing intergroup conflict.

We hoped that these meetings would increase mutual understanding of the policies, practices and operational limitations of each agency, and that cooperative procedures could be developed which would reduce tensions in the future. In turn, this increase in understanding was expected to create a more favorable organizational climate for the attitudes developed with the training sessions for policemen.

In developing that theoretical background, it has been necessary to take an ecological perspective in the sense that planned change must be considered at different levels of a social system. Interventions must be designed not only to fit the specific problems manifested at these different levels, but also to accord with the way in which these problems are interrelated. The theoretical approach presented here has applicability to a number of problems where attitudes and behavior are related to prior training, or its absence, and to experiences based on selective exposure. It is not sufficient for dealing with all types of problems, however. We felt that the group training would provide an improved baseline of attitudes and techniques, and would at the same time contribute to alleviating the problem of our visibility as consultants and increase our salience to problems in the policeman's work role. The initial approach was expected to result in an increase in the number of individual consultations requested, and in the range of problems with which help was sought.

Limitations on the levels of intervention to which we had sanctioned access, and on our time and energy as consultants, restricted the extent to which we were able to develop and employ a more complete ecological framework. Yet our awareness of the ecological perspective served to keep us alert to forces beyond our immediate arena of activity and humble in our expectations for change.

PART II

ACTIVITIES

Chapter IV

PROBLEM CONSULTATION

At times like this, I'm glad there are people like you around who I can talk to and trust.
—Spontaneous remark of policeman to consultant

W HILE THE ACTIVITIES of this entire project can be viewed as falling within a consultative framework, the content of this chapter deals with psychological consultation in the more restricted, problem-solving sense in which it has come to be used in recent literature concerning organizational development and community mental health. According to this more limited definition, consultation refers to a process in which a consultant meets with one or a group of consultees for the purpose of helping the consultees to solve some problem associated with their work roles.

As discussed in Chapter III, consultation with an individual consultee about a particular case may involve one or more of several goals. These goals are increasing the consultees' confidence, knowledge, skills, or professional objectivity. Within a consultative framework, it is also possible that the consultant will be presented with problems which are organizational or programmatic in their scope. Problems of this kind may be presented and recognized as such by the consultee, or the wider implications of discrete cases may be inferred and pointed out by the consultant. This latter interpretation of problems involves the consultant in what is variously described as administrative consultation (Caplan, 1970), or organizational consultation (Gibb and Lippitt, 1959). At this level, the consultant may be concerned with role relationships, communication patterns, and program and policy implications which effect a number of persons within an organization, as well as the clientele outside the organization.

43

A further distinction is sometimes made between the roles of consultant and consultant-trainer (Seashore and VanEgmond, 1959). The latter role differs from the former, and from that of the trainer, in that the consultant combines his or her resources as an impetus for change with continuous interaction with members of the organization in an effort to help implement new activities and to integrate changes within the on-going functions of the organization. In this role, the consultant is still an outside resource, but is more of a participant in the changes which the organization is trying to implement than would be true in either the consultant or trainer roles. This definition of the consultant-trainer role is the one which guided our activities in this project. As we conceptualized it, our role would evolve through case consultation and training to broader organizational and community concerns.

Problems and Strategies of Entry

Entry into a consultation relationship is a problem which commands ubiquitous attention from consultants and which may be regarded properly as the critical problem for this form of professional activity. While much has been written about this problem (Glidewell, 1959; Sofer, 1961; Caplan, 1970) there are a variety of contingencies influencing the strategy of the entry process. Among these factors are the nature of the initial contact, the structure and dynamics of the organization, variable perception of need within the organization, and the degree and extensity of shared goals which exist or which can be activated between the consultant and potential consultees. These concerns will also influence the subsequent course of consultation, but they are especially worthy of note in relation to how the consultant begins to work with the organization.

Organizational consultants are frequently sought by top level administrators to deal with some particular problem area which is defined organizationally from the beginning. Mental health consultants are more likely to be asked to consult with a relatively low-level problem initially, which is restricted in its organizational scope, and this contact may develop into a relationship with the organization itself. While these are the modal patterns, just the reverse may occasionally happen to each kind of consultant, of course. Regardless of the level of initial contact, it is important that the consultant establish working relationships with those levels of the organization relevant to his work and the processes involved apply to both organizational and mental health consultation. In all cases, sanction from the chief administrator will be obtained, and in many instances cooperative relationships will be sought with personnel throughout several subunits of the organization.

This project was conceived as a relatively front-line operation, and was not designed the way an organizational development model might be planned. However, we found organizational consultation concepts useful to the extent that we felt that organizational concerns would influence front-line activities and that support and understanding at all levels of the organization would be critical to the project's success. We also anticipated that in the course of the project we might be presented with concerns which were organizational in scope and we had to be prepared to deal with these as they arose.

In the initial familiarization stages of consultation, contacts will be oriented primarily towards information seeking and relationship building. The purposes sought in later contacts during the implementation phase will vary with the methods and goals of the particular type of consultation. Organizational consultants, for example, typically seek changes in the relationships between individuals or groups of consultees through group and social psychological methods. Mental health consultants who follow Caplan's case consultation framework will seek changes in the relationships of consultees to their work roles, including their clients.

The goals of the implementation phase, the expected tenure of the consultant, and the logistics of cooperation are all matters which must be agreed upon during the entry process. It is wise to keep the nature of this agreement flexible and subject to modification as new information or changing needs emerge, but it is also necessary to define some limits on the consultant's functions and to articulate an understanding of mutual responsibilities against the expectation that the consultant's role will require frequent clarification and definition and that some requests made of the consultant will be inappropriate problems for consultation.

Once these arrangements have been made, the consultant still must expect to encounter variation among consultees or groups of consultees in their accessibility and resistance to consultative activity. While the consultant has sanction to seek information from organizational personnel, consultation technique requires that potential consultees seek consultation voluntarily and remain free to accept or reject the consultant's views (Caplan, 1970). Just as there is ambiguity about what a psychologist does, there is likely to be uncertainty within the organization as to the function, purposes, and usefulness of a consultant, and this uncertainty provides opportunities to attribute a variety of motives to the consultant which may or may not fit the consultant's role. The structure and dynamics of the organization will have a more proximal effect on the flow of information to potential consultees about the consultant's presence and goals. The sources and methods of communication of this information may effect the way in which this information is interpreted and the purposes with which potential consultees may approach the consultant (Mann, 1972). The experienced consultant can use these phenomena to pose hypotheses about the nature of the organization and the needs of individual members.

Additionally, both as a function of organizational role and individual characteristics, consultees will vary in their awareness of the need for change. For example, an individual who is highly invested in a particular method of functioning and who receives little feedback as to its effectiveness from the standpoint of the organization's goals, or who receives positive feedback in terms of personal goals which may vary from those of the organization, will be unlikely to perceive a need for change. Similarly, individuals with little expectation for change, because of past frustrations, cynicism, or a lack of involvement in their job, such as those who may be merely putting in their time waiting for retirement, will perceive little need for change. Such persons may see the consultant as a threat to the *status quo,* or as an agent of the top administrator who has been sent in to *shake up the troops.*

Others may see themselves as the target of change and may view the consultant as an opportunity to bootleg some psychotherapy or as an intrusion to be avoided lest they reveal their own perceived inadequacies. The combined mythology surrounding mental health professionals and the uncertainty associated with the role of the consultant will likely arouse some of these motivations in most people, and they are problems with which the consultant must deal by seeking coordinate, collaborative relationships, by clearly and repeatedly articulating his role, and by seeking agreement as to goals.

In pursuing the definition of goals which can be shared between consultant and consultee, the consultant must also be aware of the nonobvious sources from which goals may arise. On the one hand, the consultant must be alert to the possibility that he may impose his own agenda in ways which conflict with the aims of the consultees. On the other hand, he must recognize those goals of individual consultees and of the consultee system which may be legitimate, but which are latent and unarticulated during the entry process, and accommodate these in setting explicit goals. Among the former may be values associated with the consultant's profession, such as openness, flexibility and a preference for intellectualization over action which may or may not be appropriate to the consultees' work roles. The latter might include concerns for personal status and security and the protection and enhancement of the public image of the consultee system. These issues demand consideration in any consultation setting, of course, and they are probably not as secret as some observers might believe. Whether or not they need to be made explicit, and the degree to which they need to be examined, should depend on the purpose such explication will serve in furthering other goals. Frequently these issues will surface anyway as the relationship between consultant and consultees develops, and the consultant's primary concern is that they not be thwarted in fact or in appearance during early planning.

The reader will recall that Chapters I and II traced the sequence of the entry process. At this point examination of the reasoning behind the sequence, and the development of further opportunities for consultation, can be provided through examples of consultation problems which will serve to relate this aspect of the project to the preceding discussion as well as to the other activities of the consultants.

The Consultant Role

The Psychological Consultation project grew directly from the response of policemen to the psychology course taught by the author for members of the police department (Mann, 1970) in that several policemen voiced the wish that the author could be available to discuss practical aspects of their work as they occurred. This overture was pursued by some key members of the department who were interested in the professional development of the police role in general, and in the educational development of the personnel in their department in particular, through several discussions with the author. A written proposal was developed, discussed and modified, and submitted to the Chief of Police for further discussion. After this review and additional modifications, the proposal was presented to the department's Training Committee, composed of key staff and supervisory personnel representing the various components of the organization. These deliberations provided an opportunity for participation in planning the project by personnel at different levels and from each operational unit of the department which led eventually to the submission of a grant request from the department to the Hogg Foundation for Mental Health for support of the two-year demonstration period.

As a consequence of the psychology course, attended by personnel from virtually every level of the department, the author had established some form of relationship with several persons in the organization. As the nature of the relationship was transformed into a consultative one, several problems related to the entry process had to be solved. First, the deliberations with the chief and his staff culminating in the submission of the grant request from the police department was necessary to achieve official sanction and to define the project as belonging to the department rather than the consultant. Second, it was necessary to redefine the author's relationship to the department from that of teacher to that of consultant. This redefinition was a continuous process throughout the project for various personnel in the organization, and was aided by frequent advice and feedback from members of the department, without whose help the process would have been exceedingly difficult.

Case Consultation

The consultant team composed of the supervising consultant and student consultants from the Community Mental Health Training Program at the University of Texas, faced the problem of deploying themselves so as to be maximally visible and appropriately available for individual consultations. Initially, the team visited the department in a group during the familiarization phase so that the student consultants could acquire the benefits of the supervising consultant's existing relationships. On completion of this phase, each consultant was physically present in the department for one-half day each week. Problems of space precluded the consultants from having an identifiable office location, making it necessary for the consultants to adopt a *floating* routine in which they tried to be present in key areas of interaction.

After being introduced in a group during the *show-up* or assembly period prior to the beginning of each shift, the consultants made it a practice to attend these sessions when they were present in the department. In addition, the consultants made a point of *checking in* regularly with certain offices. These included the Community Relations Office, the Captain of Police Office, where the officer in charge of each shift is located; the Homicide Detail of the Criminal Investigation Division, and the Training Office of the Service Division. This routine was initiated by the consultants for the purpose of seeking information from the personnel in each of these offices about the kind of problems which they considered to be most significant and the ways in which they thought consultation might be helpful.

Both the physical and social arrangements of the various settings seemed to contribute to the number and kind of consultation problems which were presented. During the show-up periods, there were occasional requests for general information from the consultant in regard to special cases with which everyone on that shift might become concerned, such as reports of mental hospital escapes or complaints which had been received about an especially disturbing individual for whom the police were to be alerted. More often, however, patrolmen who did seek consultative help would do so in a hallway before or after the show-up period, and then seemingly almost by accident. Still, in proportion to the number of men involved, consultation requests from and around the show-up setting were never as frequent as those arising from the other settings, and proportionately more requests came from personnel in the office settings we visited frequently.

From the perspective of Lewin's field of forces concept (1951), this effect may be interpreted as consistent with the hypothesis that in a larger group, the forces acting on any given individual will be less than in a small group. According to this view, policemen in the larger group represented by the show-up setting would feel less need to approach the consultants, while in less populated settings such as offices and hallways these forces would operate more strongly on individuals. An analogous effect has been proposed by Latane and Darley (reported by Wheeler, 1970) to explain the lack of response of bystanders to an emergency. They suggest that there is a diffusion of responsibility when there are several onlookers. This diffusion effect however, accounts for only part of the behavior observed in such situations. Other variables may counteract or increase the intensity of the forces operating in such situations, as Latane and Darley recognized in their experiments.

In the case of the show-up setting, there were very probably strong social norms operating against contact with the consultant. One very common source of resistance is simply the on-going patterns of social interaction among the members of a shift which have been established and reinforced in previous experience and do not readily provide a role for a newcomer (See Chapter XI). Another factor could be a group norm about presenting a public image of rugged self-reliance in regard to work-role functions, which might especially affect young patrolmen eager to establish themselves in the eyes of their peers, during the show-up period, and a consequent reluctance to appear in need of help by approaching the consultant.

Other explanations could also be advanced. There are institutionalized procedures for seeking advice or guidance from members of one's shift, including peers and supervisors, which would meet some of an individual's needs for such help and may serve to define and limit the kinds of problems for which guidance is sought in a way in which consultation with an outside resource would not be seen as relevant. Moreover, to the extent that policemen learn about their job from other policemen through a kind of social comparison process (Mann, 1971), a consultant would not provide the degree of similarity to the policeman, which is thought to be an important incentive for social comparison, that other policemen would represent. In this context, consultant-consultee differences in socioeconomic background and a tendency to see the consultant as an intimidating expert would be included as impediments to seeking consultation. While these latter factors can account for the cohesiveness which exists among a given group of police officers assigned to the same shift, the explanation cannot account for the contacts with the consultants outside of the show-up setting without some *ad hoc* propositions to account for this contradictory behavior. The more inclusive field-of-forces concept seems to provide a more useful level of conceptualization, within which such factors as help-seeking habits and social comparison processes can be included as forces.

While this theoretical excursion may seem to be a digression, we found that such exercises frequently led to clarification of the course of our work and led us to modify our practices in ways which promised to be more productive. For example, within the field-of-forces framework, additional findings in the experiments conducted by Latane and Darley suggested some heuristic possibilities for both our theory and practices. Their experiments concerned the responsiveness of observers to apparent victims. They found that by providing prior acquaintance between observers and victims, the diffusion of responsibility effects could be eliminated; that is, personal acquaintance increased the forces operating on the observer to respond. While we did not see ourselves as *victims,* and the policemen need not have felt any responsibility to seek consultation, the principle of increasing attraction forces through prior acquaintance would seem to apply equally well to the consultation process.

Applied to this particular consultation problem we sought to increase our familiarity with policemen through the other activities described in this report on the assumption that this would eventually increase the frequency with which consultation would be sought on a problem-centered basis. Some partial support for this assumption was obtained from the fact that we were approached for consultation more frequently by those patrolmen with whom we had ridden in the Buddy System.

Still, the overall number of consultation requests arising among patrolmen was disappointingly small, and our opportunities for increasing acquaintance with a large number of patrolmen were limited by their being dispersed individually outside of the assembly setting. It seemed more efficient to seek acquaintance with patrolmen in group settings where mental health issues were more central and where counteracting social forces would be reduced.

This limited sampling of consultation contacts also affected the kinds of problems presented for consultation, varieties of which will be discussed in more detail subsequently. Most of the problem cases presented in this context were of a chronic, relatively insoluble, but at the same time not terribly pressing and acute, nature, and in pursuing these cases diagnostically we encountered more problems of lack of knowledge, skill and confidence than of theme interference.

We began to regard the order of consultee problems presented by Caplan (1970, p. 127) as approximating a kind of hierarchy analogous to the need hierarchy proposed in Maslow's (1943) theory of personality. In this case the sequence would correspond to a course of professional development rather than the broader scope of personal history. We were working with a consultee system in which most members had not achieved a professional level of competence in dealing with problems of mental health; indeed, that was the reason for our planning to participate in structured training activities. While the original plan called for simultaneous training and case consultation, we began to believe that, with the resources at our command, it would be more efficient to look at these activities sequentially. Caplan has reached a somewhat similar conclusion in the preface to his book, indicating that some organizations require a more developmental approach before they are ready to take full advantage of consultation activities:

"They ask for a consultant, but they need someone who will combine consultation with straight-forward teaching, supervision, and collaboration—someone who will "pitch in and get his hands dirty." (1970, xii)

The hierarchical conception of consultation needs was reinforced by our experience that we received proportionately more frequent and more meaningful consultation requests from those policemen who had specialized training and were more mature and sophisticated, regardless of years of experience.

Accordingly, we decided that a shift in emphasis was in order which would increase our involvement in training activities. Our concerns and proposals were presented to the Training Committee during a periodic review of the project. They expressed concern that more case consultation problems were not being presented and began to explore with us ways of increasing our utilization. However, they also agreed that the shift in emphasis was appropriate. These discussions had two consequences. One was to provide larger blocks of time in the training program for the activities which we proposed. The other was the beginning of a continuing examination of some of the social forces among the patrol organizations related to our project.

In conducting other activities we were still present physically to handle those consultation requests which did occur and were making more economical use of our resources. We continued to attend the show-up meetings occasionally, but not as religiously as we had done at first. In making this shift, we anticipated that there would be an increase in demand for case consultation at which time we could alter our strategy again. Unfortunately, the time span of the demonstration period was too short to provide an appropriate test of this assumption, since it would require an interval sufficient to allow a significant number of personnel who had more structured acquaintance with us in training settings to pass on through a period of job experience in which new approaches could be tried and questioned before an increase in consultation requests would be expected.

We were also limiting seriously the chances of obtaining significant measurable changes during this time period, but this probably would have been true regardless of whether or not we had shifted emphasis, given the conditions which existed. It did indicate that we would have to look for more changes among those groups with whom we had conducted training activities than those with whom we had case consultation experiences.

Examples of Case Consultation Problems

The kinds of cases presented initially were consistent with our experience in other settings, and with the experience of other consultants, that the first problems about which consultation is sought tend to be those which have frustrated the consultee system for some time. By virtue of this history of contact, consultees have often developed some routine ways of managing such cases, and it cannot be assumed readily that these routines are inappropriate. It is necessary to examine each case not only from the standpoint of what should be done in some abstract sense, but also as to what can or cannot be done realistically in view of the resources available.

The most frequent problem case was what we came to call *the lonely little old lady* syndrome. These consisted of older persons living alone who called persistently to report prowlers, thieves, or occasionally visitors from outer space, on their property. When investigated, even the first two kinds of intruders were never present and the complaints were unfounded in reality. It is departmental policy that all complaints are investigated by officers in person and communications center personnel do not intervene with such callers. Thus, officers were asked to respond to situations where they had probably had similar complaints previously and since they believed the complaint to be unfounded before the fact they considered these assignments a waste of time, and sought consultation in hopes of achieving some relief.

As consultants, our first question in response to such cases was to inquire about past practices and results. We discovered a range of creative responses which varied in their effectiveness. Most policemen assumed that such persons were having delusions or hallucinations, although they did not label them as such. In *the old days* officers might fire a couple of shots in the air out of sight of the complainant and then report to them that the intruder had been killed. Others would thank the complainant for the information, which they said pertained to an important case on which they were working and which they would now be able to solve. Still others would try to talk to the person about things which might be worrying them. The persistence of these complaints suggested that such solutions were relatively ineffective.

These cases may be viewed as examples of partial social and sensory deprivation in which the complainant's experiences arose out of limited opportunities for consensually validating their perceptions. Their persistent responses, which almost always occurred during late evening or early morning hours, could be seen as means by which the complainants were seeking attention and companionship, as well as a corroboration of their experiences. Some policemen recognized this element of the situation, too. One reported that he was able to reduce the frequency of calling in a chronic case by telling the complainant that he would keep a watch for intruders, and then would drive past the complainant's house periodically and flash his red light as a signal that he was keeping his word. Others would alert relatives, if there were any available, to make more frequent contacts with the complainants.

As a group, these calls represent a problem in social resources. While the policemen considered such calls as nuisances, by serving as a meaningful social contact they were providing a useful service to the complaining parties. Unfortunately, as is true with most such human service tasks, since the policemen were not rewarded in any way for these activities, it was difficult to see them as being worthwhile.

By defining the problem in social terms, these calls can be seen as a symptom of a failure of community social organization, one of many such symptoms which fall to the police for handling by default. The question then becomes one of defining appropriate social solutions. The simplest solution would be to mobilize family or companionship resources, as some policemen correctly did. However, not all such cases have family or friends immediately available. In these instances, some form of substitute social contact seems necessary. Since few social agencies operate 24-hours-a-day, the police will probably continue to play an important social function with such persons. Our immediate task was to try to change the definition of these situations so that they could be more rewarding psychologically to policemen by helping them understand the social implications of this kind of activity. A more long term response would be to change the definition of police work to include these and many similar instances of human intervention for which policemen receive little or no official recognition. Short of redefining in some supersocietal way the nature of the responsibilities of family, neighbors, and other potential social resources toward a variety of socially isolated persons, this arrangement seems preferable to implementing a bureaucratic social service program to meet the needs of people who paradoxically might see such a program as an unwarranted intrusion of their privacy.

The second most frequent case was what might be called the *multi-agency adolescent*. In one case, we received three separate requests for consultation from different policemen on the same youth. Typically, these cases involved a complicated and disorganized family structure out of which an adolescent had become involved in a long history of contact with social agencies, police, and courts for deviant behavior. The police contact was usually after the fact in that a pattern of deviant behavior which had defied social agency solution was well established. In some cases, the youth and his family were known personally to the policeman, and he sought advice as to how he could be helpful to the boy on an unofficial basis, such as by trying to establish a friendship.

These cases raise a number of issues. Most policemen thought of such cases as opportunities for prevention, by which they meant prevention of an adult criminal career. Yet, from the standpoint of mental health prevention, most such cases were beyond the point of anything short of a tertiary preventive effort. One would ordinarily think of improving interagency coordination in such cases to achieve better tertiary prevention, although during the course of the project at least, such youth seemed capable of acting out to the point of being faced with criminal charges faster than the agencies could achieve coordination. The policeman's interest in preventive work could be an important primary preventive force, yet those officers who spent much time befriending youth who were not already in trouble were vulnerable to the suspicion that they were wasting time which should be spent on other pursuits from officers within the department to whom they were accountable. Once again, the issue of reward structure and role definition asserts its salience, but better prevention could be achieved by utilizing this motivation of policemen before the fact.[7]

A second issue raised by these cases is the question of coordination among policemen within the department. The fact that these cases had multiple contact within the department was seldom checked out by patrolmen, although the information was contained in the police files. Often these previous reports contained important family history or agency contact information which might not be obtained from the subject in subsequent contacts, and which could be useful in more efficient handling of such cases. A specialized section of police record keeping and information retrieval for juvenile cases might pay dividends in better efficiency.

Encountering such refractive cases in the initial phases of mental health consultation is often frustrating to novice or student consultants, and there is an understandable impulse on their part to quickly define the problem as insoluble from the consultee's standpoint and to encourage the consultee to do likewise. Yet, such cases can serve a useful introductory function for the consultant. For one thing, they provide information about the problems of community services in general and the consultee's organization in particular which is disproportionate to their number, since such cases are usually over-representative from the standpoint of social agency contacts. For another, they provide an excellent avenue for the consultant to begin to explore for theme interferences which may have some generality within the consultee system. Telling the consultee merely that such cases are difficult to handle will not come exactly as a great revelation to

---

[7] The concepts of prevention used here follow the public health practice of classifying prevention into three levels. Primary prevention refers to efforts to reduce the incidence, or first occurrence, of problems; secondary prevention means attempts to reduce the severity of problems and the likelihood of more serious ones developing; and tertiary prevention deals with trying the reduce the chronicity of problems by mediating or eliminating the social after-effects of a severe problem (Brown, 1961).

him, and since exploration of the case provides an opportunity for the consultant to demonstrate his operational method to the consultee, these cases should not be considered a waste of time. Some of the novice consultant's apprehension about such cases may arise from a lack of clarity as to what is expected of him at this point. It is more important that he demonstrate his willingness to examine the case openly and thoroughly, to explore the consultee's past efforts and future alternatives, and to honestly admit his own limitations, than it is for him to demonstrate his ability to produce instant success. Clear definition of the consultant role at this point should produce more meaningful consultations in the future, while too much initial success might establish unrealistic expectations or reduce the consultee's motivation for seeking further consultation.

In fact, the kinds of problems presented for consultation in this project did show a progression towards more susceptibility to successful intervention. In the area of case consultation, there were increasing requests to review with policemen the effects of alternative behaviors on their part on the course and outcome of family disputes, handling of abusive and potentially assaultive subjects, and interactions with members of groups which were salient to police work but not specifically involved in criminal events, such as youth and members of the university fringe community, the street people.

There was also an increasing number of requests for consultation on intraorganizational concerns. Among these were issues related to supervision and assignment of personnel, communication and morale problems within organizational units of the department, and the planning and development of the Police-Community Relations program. A significant amount of time was also spent on problems of personnel recruitment and selection, which deserves some further discussion.

Personnel Selection

The issue of selecting potential policemen is both complex and important, and has received extensive attention from both police administrators and behavioral scientists. There are several excellent references on the subject which examine the issues more thoroughly than our involvement in the problem in this project would justify.[8] The limited degree to which we became involved in this problem was dictated more by other demands than by the importance of selection procedures.

The average citizen is probably only minimally aware of the criteria involved in selecting candidates for police work or of the qualifications of those who survive the process. Yet, among police administrators and the public alike, there persists a wish to make the personnel selection process even more effective, particularly in assessing psychological suitability. Communities insist, rightly, that those who are given official sanction to use coercive force (Bittner, 1970) as part of their work be scrutinized carefully against possible personal tendencies to misuse this sanction. In this particular department, three procedures were used to detect such tendencies. Each candidate was required to take the Minnesota Multiphasic Personality Inventory (MMPI), a thorough background investigation was conducted, and candidates were examined in a stress-interview by an oral interview board of police supervisory personnel. The author was asked to interpret the MMPI profiles of applicants and report his impressions as part of the screening process.

Prior to making interpretations, it was stipulated and agreed that impressions from the MMPI profile could not serve as a basis for selection by themselves. Therefore, the interpretations were directed toward suggesting areas for further investigation, either in the background investigation or by the oral interview board. It was also suggested that the use of the MMPI and other tests be subjected to systematic research, but this was not undertaken during the course of the project.

While the feedback which the author received on his interpretations was encouraging, the process of reviewing numerous profiles was extremely time-consuming, and it seemed questionable whether the unknown utility of the reports justified the investment of time and effort. Moreover, the author had to consider

---

[8] Niederhoffer (1967, Chapter 2) lists the major references to this topic. Other important references include the *Task Force Report: The Police,* President's Commission on Law Enforcement and Administration of Justice (1967), and Rhead, *et al.,* (1968).

how the interpretive process would be conducted beyond his tenure as a consultant. The possibility of using computerized interpretations was explored by submitting some sample profiles and comparing interpretations as to utility of content. This comparison indicated that the computerized interpretations provided sufficient information for screening purposes, and since they were more economical and did not depend on the availability of the consultant, it was decided to begin using the computer interpretation services. There remains, however, a need to explore this area systematically so that interpretations, which are currently made from the standpoint of general personality functioning, could be made more pertinent to the selection of police candidates in particular. Moreover, this activity resulted only in improved efficiency of the existing selection procedure, which should not be confused with an improvement in the accuracy of the selection procedure itself. The latter would require an extensive program of psychometric investigation.

Crisis Consultation

Crisis situations in the form of events for which an organization is unprepared or which threaten to overwhelm the response capacities of an organization even in the face of some anticipation can be significant milestones in the development of an organization's operational patterns. These events require rapid, innovative decisions to be made which can effect, proactively or reactively, the organization's handling of future situations. Within Caplan's consultative framework, crisis situations are thought to especially ripen opportunities for consultative intervention. Such an opportunity arose during the course of the project, and it proved to be a critical event in fostering a working relationship between the department and the consultants.

The widespread student protests following the United States' invasion of Cambodia occurred about midway through the project's demonstration period. Austin and the University of Texas campus were no exceptions to this phenomenon, but the course of events was significantly different from that which took place in some cities. This event was also the only protest demonstration of significant and potentially dangerous magnitude which has occurred in the city during this age of protest and unrest. Despite its novelty, the concerted efforts of numerous groups and individuals were eventually successful in bringing to a peaceful conclusion a situation which seemed at times to promise disaster.

During this week of tension and uncertainty, we were in the fortuitous position of being able to offer services to the Police Department and to be participant observers in events on the campus and in the community. In addition to providing consultation to the Police Department regarding the events which were developing, we were able to provide liaison with other significant groups involved. The details of these activities have been reported elsewhere (Mann and Iscoe, 1971), but it is important to point out here the advantages of having an established working relationship between behavioral scientists and a major behavior-controlling institution which can be mobilized during crisis situations such as the Cambodian demonstrations. The quality of that relationship is illustrated by the quotation which appears at the beginning of this chapter, a comment which was made as the peaceful parade of demonstrators neared its conclusion.

These working relationships repay the time and effort involved in establishing them several-fold during crisis events, while it is difficult if not impossible to develop the same quality of cooperation at the time a crisis occurs. Moreover, the successful management of critical situations become a matter of justifiable organizational pride which reflects in further developments in the working relationship. While the exact timing of crisis situations cannot be predicted, the probability of their occurrence in some form can be anticipated.

From the vantage point of reflection, it is especially clear that an open-ended developmental time perspective is essential to the conduct of community intervention programs. That is, while there are explicit relatively short-term changes which intervention programs hope to accomplish, there are also continually changing needs which organizations and communities face, not all of which can be anticipated at the outset of a change program. Therefore, an important goal of consultative activities should be to promote changes which will serve not only immediate ends, but which will also prepare the client system for enhanced coping with unanticipated future events.

In this context, the activities described in this report can be viewed as efforts to accomplish the establishment and testing of a working relationship which will have, hopefully, continuing future benefits. For example, the strategies outlined here which involved the deliberate manipulation of the relationship between consultation, training, and community organization activities were designed to change the way in which the members of the organization are able to make use of outside resources. In addition, by setting a precedent for cooperation between policemen and *outside intellectuals,* a process has been initiated which may be generalized to productive relationships with others who can make a contribution to the improved conduct of community life through the police organization.

Along this same line, it is necessary for the consultant to plan his activities so that the change-oriented procedures which he implements will become eventually a self-sustaining part of the organization's functioning. As we pursued this line of thinking, we were able to see specific opportunities for deliberately influencing the social-psychological processes of the department so as to enhance its sense of *ownership* of the project and increase the probability of the activities becoming self-sustaining. A specific example of this kind of process was a special training program in which we planned to train police officers to provide training for other policemen in stress experiences designed to influence social norms within the department. In this activity, we were involved in consulting with the prospective trainer within the department.

Stress Training

The medium for this training activity was a set of three films, *The Police Experience Film Modules,* distributed under the auspices of the International Association of Chiefs of Police. Each film deals with a set of emotions commonly encountered in police work, *Fear and Anxiety, Feeling Good,* and *Humiliation and Anger.* The films run for ten minutes or less, and depict policemen encountering situations which are quite powerful in eliciting the respective emotional reactions. Interspersed throughout the enactment of each situation are comments from police officers expressing their own emotional reactions to the events portrayed, and to the actions of policemen in handling the situations. The films serve as a springboard for extended discussion during which policemen have the opportunity to express their emotional reactions, to share these reactions with fellow policemen, and to explore the basis for them and the relationship of emotions to actions. From a social-psychological standpoint, the films provide an opportunity to influence social comparison processes among policemen in relation to crisis situations which are thought to be important determinants of informal social norms governing policemen's behavior in emotion-laden events (Mann, 1971).

At our suggestion, the department purchased the films which were then reviewed and demonstrated for command-level personnel. In this context, the expected reservations which some officers had about the films were discussed and an agreement was reached as to their use. It was decided that a member of the consultation team would conduct the initial training sessions jointly with an experienced police officer, with the understanding the policeman would eventually be able to conduct the training sessions himself and could in turn train other officers to conduct them. While this was an important ingredient from the standpoint of future use of this training experience it was especially appropriate because of the delicacy involved in policemen discussing their emotional reactions with each other. We felt that this process would be facilitated if the trainer were a policeman himself.

In addition to whatever changes this program might produce in individual policemen or in the social norms related to crisis situations, we hoped that these training experiences might make the public discussion of emotionally charged situations more acceptable among the policemen, which would in turn decrease the social forces operating against their seeking help in dealing with crises in the community, either from consultants or their fellow officers. Once again, however, the expected realization of these goals extends beyond the duration of the demonstration project.

These efforts may be considered analogous to the planting of seeds of possibilities which may come to fruition later through the efforts of the members of the Police Department and the community to continue their nurturance and development. At this point, we can only hope to satisfy ourselves that we have succeeded in germinating a hardy variety of ideas. After some further discussion of our activities in training and promoting interagency cooperation, we can return to a consideration of the evidence of how these initial efforts may have succeeded.

Chapter V

TRAINING

The three of us attended one afternoon session of a week-long workshop in leadership training at the Police Association Building. About fifteen persons from a cross-section of supervisory levels attended. We were introduced and invited to participate in the discussion regarding the problem exercises on which they were working. However, it was apparent that we were to be set off from the rest. We were seated three in a row in a corner of the room, which made me feel apart, *looked at,* and uncomfortable. A few kidding comments directed at us soon made it apparent that we were to be viewed as the *panel of experts* who had the *right* answers. We each made a few remarks on various cases, then explained our project to them in some detail. In this meeting we thus shared a little of our personalities with them and communicated intellectually about our project. Still, it was apparent that we had a very long way to go in establishing individual rapport with them.

—Notes from a student consultant's log

THE TRAINING ACTIVITIES to be discussed in this chapter are presented in roughly the chronological order in which they occurred. While other activities are described in subsequent chapters, it is important for the reader to keep in mind that we were simultaneously involved in consulting with members of the police department about other matters as they occurred and in organizing and conducting the series of interagency meetings described previously. As the student consultant's remarks indicate, it was necessary to establish and maintain relationships with numerous people in the department, and to demonstrate our commitment to dealing with real problems if we were to go beyond our initial image of *experts.*

This problem is intimately related to the process of influencing behavior. Using a theoretical framework developed by French and Raven (1959), Bennis (1966) notes that consultants frequently enter an organization on the basis of their expert power, but their more important influence stems from their success in acquiring referent power. This concept implies that the consultees are influenced by their liking for the change agent, as distinct from their respect for his expertise.

The training system of the department had its own structure, personnel and norms, and it was necessary to plan our entry just as with any other system. Our approach was to serve as resource personnel for existing training activities, and as needs for additional training activities were articulated, to develop and conduct them.

Our first contact with the training system was in the leadership training session for supervisors referred to above. This served as a convenient introduction to a sample of the supervisory personnel, but did not represent a significant training activity for the project. Supervisory training could have been a significant part of the project, but no activities for this purpose were conducted during the period covered by this report. Additional comments on training for supervisory personnel will be found in the chapter on organizational structure. With two exceptions, formalized training activities were confined to police cadets.

The Cadet Training Program

The Austin Police Cadets receive 20 weeks of training, meeting five days per week for classroom and practical problem sessions, and one day per week for practical experience, accompanying an experienced officer. In addition to learning about laws, departmental policies and practical techniques of traditional law enforcement activities, the cadets receive specialized training in community relations, family disturbances, disasters, and demonstrations and social protests. At the time the project began, the only specific training dealing with mentally disturbed behavior was the practical problem described in the previous chapter, and an annual one-day workshop sponsored by the Austin-Travis County Mental Health Association.

Extensive use of the *practical problem* method of training was employed. Problem situations were selected by the instructors which illustrated an important point of law, policy, or procedure, or all of these factors. Instructors role-played the subjects involved with a great deal of realism, and it must be admitted the deck was usually stacked against the cadet handling the situation successfully. Cadets were assigned to handle these problems in turns in front of their classmates. After each presentation, the situation was discussed by both instructors and cadets, and then repeated several times. On successive repetitions, the behavior of the intructors was varied somewhat to maintain the element of surprise and prevent the development of mechanical procedures by the cadets.

In order to integrate ourselves into this system, we began by observing training sessions and participating in the discussions which followed the problems. We were able to learn along with the cadets about the legal, policy and procedural constraints and alternatives operating on their behavior in such situations, and thus could make contributions which were both appropriate and consistent with the policeman's required operational patterns. After participating in the training of one cadet class in this way, we were asked increasingly to make recommendations for and to participate in modifications and additions to the training program. As we did so, and as our relationships within the department progressed, our activities were accepted as an integral part of the program.

Community Relations

Our first invitation to suggest modifications in training came after attending a session on police-community relations called Project Understanding. The purpose of the training was to expose the police cadets to individuals from the community who talked about problems which they perceived in police-community relations. In the morning, high school students composed the community representation, and in the afternoon adults from the community participated. The format of these discussions had the community representatives seated at a table in the front of the room, with the police cadets seated in a group facing them. Each member of the community *panel* was asked to make a statement about some experience they had had with policemen, and then these were discussed. Police instructors served as moderators, asking questions of the panel, and clarifying issues of law and policy which arose from the panelists' remarks.

The tone of these discussions was highly controlled, with the community members, particularly the high school students, appearing somewhat intimidated and restrained. The physical arrangement, both the positioning and the distance between the groups, inhibited close personal exchanges, and the majority of exchanges took place between the citizens and the instructor-moderators who were seated closer to the panelists. Both the cadets and the instructors expressed dissatisfaction with the arrangement and asked for our suggestions for improvement.

In addition to the physical factors described above, there were other factors which seemed to prevent a basically good idea from achieving its potential. The community representatives seemed to have been highly selected, either by accident or design, to represent a rather narrow sample in what was in fact a diverse community. High school principals tended to select their *best citizens* as representatives, and while the adult panelists contained some minority group members, the range of attitudes and opinions represented was not typical of these groups in the community.

On the other hand, we learned that in the past the police had experienced a narrow selection of community members in the other direction, that is representatives among the adult panelists who were extremely hostile to the police. The police perceived these persons as unrepresentative and irresponsible, with effects which tended to limit exchanges in ways similar to those described above.

Perhaps because of this experience, and/or for other reasons, the instructor-moderators in these sessions were at some pains to insure that police department policy and legal implications were clearly and fully articulated in relation to each incident discussed. This practice, however, placed them in a position of intervening rather frequently in the discussions and further limiting spontaneity. While we respected the necessity of such clarifications, the end result was more understanding of the police by the citizens than understanding of the community by the cadets.

We felt that the cadets could probably handle most issues of law and policy by this stage of their training, at least to the extent that was necessary in these sessions, and that the goals of achieving more informal and personal understandings with the community were more important to the cadets than the public relations and community education gains which could be made in this format.

Accordingly, we suggested a format in which more representative community members would be involved, both from the high school and adult populations, in order to broaden the attitudinal sample to which the cadets were exposed. In turn, this meant that the Police Department would have to establish or activate relationships with representative segments of the community in order to solicit the participation of such persons. This latter point was not a primary goal, however, since there are more effective means of achieving such relationships than through this program.[9]

We also suggested changing the physical arrangement of the program, so that a few cadets would sit in a group with two or three of the community representatives, thus equalizing the social forces operating on members of both groups and promoting more personal exchanges. Further, we suggested employing moderators who were skilled in group discussion techniques in order to facilitate group interaction. Persons who performed this function in subsequent training sessions were the student consultants, professional psychologists in the community, and a minister on the faculty of a local seminary who was experienced in group work.

In order to implement the strategy of loosening stereotypes prior to exposure, a one-hour introductory session was held with the cadets some days prior to the group discussions. This session consisted of a brief lecture by the author on the psychology of person perception, and how people use superficial and often irrelevant cues to make judgment of others. The lecture was followed by an exercise in which the cadets were asked to imagine a man walking down the street with long hair, wearing a buckskin suit with beads around his neck. With no more information than this, they were asked to state what inferences they could make about him. The responses of the cadets were listed on a chalk-board.

These instructions produced a number of inferred judgments,

---

[9] Such relationships did in fact exist, and others have been established through the Department's active Police-Community Relations Program.

ranging from an "individualistic non-conformist" through an "anti-American hippy-type" to a "potential thief or burglar" (the latter based on the assumption that the individual was probably a drug user and would steal to support his habits). After several such stereotyped responses had been produced, the cadets were told that the person whom the author had in mind in describing this individual was Jay Silverheels, the Indian film and television actor, and he happened to be in town in connection with a movie he had made.

The exercise was followed by further discussion of the fallacies of relying on superficial appearance in making judgments, and the necessity of trying to seek more reliable information through personal acquaintance in making such judgments. While they could all see the difference between their initial impressions and the kind of evidence they would need to substantiate their impressions, the cadets reported that this was a dramatic illustration for them of the role of stereotyped thinking.

The groups were given problem topics as spring boards for discussion, and the moderators attempted to elicit personal reactions and experiences from the group members as the discussion progressed. After an hour's discussion, each group selected a member to report the gist of their deliberations to the other groups, and a general discussion followed. Then the participants changed groups and discussed a new problem. At the end of the second discussion, the community representatives were replaced by a new group of citizens and additional problem discussions were conducted.

These changes produced obvious and immediate differences in the degree of participation and level of intensity of the discussions. The feedback from cadets, instructors and community participants was highly favorable. In addition, these sessions led to important unanticipated consequences which pointed out the need for additional activities in police-community relations. Some of the high school students were impressed with their contacts with the police cadets, and felt that further contact between the cadets and their fellow students would be mutually beneficial. They invited the cadets to visit their schools and meet with other students and took the initiative in making the arrangements. The invitation was accepted enthusiastically. These changes were then adopted as part of the training program and employed with succeeding cadet classes.

Training in Interviews

The Criminal Investigation Division requested training in interview techniques for their personnel, which would include an emphasis on sensitivity to interpersonal nuances as well as a means of obtaining information. The interview is a major technique for CID personnel in relating to complainants, persons seeking information, lost or neglected children, emotionally disturbed persons, and others, as well as witnesses and subjects in criminal investigation.

We observed interviews conducted by CID personnel with a variety of subjects in different settings and designed a training session which applied our knowledge and style of interviewing to their particular needs. All members of the division attended one of two half-day sessions.

Each trainee was given an outline of basic interviewing principles and techniques[10] which was discussed by the consultants. This was followed by a presentation on the process of inference from interview observations, including non-verbal cues, the effects of the interviewer's behavior on the interviewee, and the effects of cultural and life style differences between interviewer and subject on the interview process. Tape recordings of interviews were played along with comments and questions directed to the trainees illustrating points in the preceding discussion. Finally, several interview situations were role-played with trainees taking the roles of interviewer and interviewee. The alter-ego technique was employed in which other trainees were asked to observe either interviewer or interviewee silently and try to imagine the effect of the other person's behavior on their particular subject. At the end of the role-playing, participants and alter-egos discussed and compared their reactions to the situation.

While no particular effort was made to evaluate this training session systematically,[11] it was gratifying to observe the techniques

---

[10] Constructed by David Hopkinson.

[11] At the end of each training session, participants were asked to write down their reactions and suggestions for improvement. These responses were nearly unanimously favorable, but do not reflect meaningfully the effects of the training.

discussed being employed by CID personnel on at least some occasions. One such event which is memorable was the sight of several CID personnel employing the principle of literally and physically getting down to the subject's level when interviewing children. Several policemen were observed squatting at eye-level around a small, lost girl in an effort to ascertain her identity and find out where she lived. Although we had always observed the policemen to be friendly and solicitous of small children in such circumstances, we had not seen this particular technique employed prior to the training session.[12]

Mental Health Problems

An opportunity to become involved with training in handling disturbed behavior arose from our being asked to help in planning the annual workshop sponsored by the Mental Health Association near the end of our familiarization phase. In the past, several formats had been employed in these one-day sessions, and while policemen felt the workshops had been helpful, they also felt there was room for improvement in providing information which was more meaningful for police work. It was felt that we could provide this kind of input because of our familiarity with police work and our knowledge of behavior.

We saw the workshop format as a potential prototype of the interagency meetings we hoped to conduct, but we also felt that the workshop could at best be only supplementary to other specific training in assessment and intervention with the mentally disturbed. We agreed to help organize the workshop, but we also requested and received time in the cadet training schedule for activities of the latter kind.

Design of the training program for mental health problems followed the theoretical analysis presented in Chapter III. The training sessions began with a brief lecture presentation of the main types and behavior patterns of mental disorders, placing special emphasis on those behavioral features which would prob-

---

[12] This and other techniques in interviewing children are presented in Newman and Keith (1964).

ably be apparent to the policeman encountering such behavior on the street. The cadets' attention was also directed to the small booklet for policemen on recognizing and handling disturbed behavior published by the National Association for Mental Health (Matthews and Rowland, 1964) which was available in the Police Department Library.

After questions and discussion of the lecture material, the cadets participated in role-playing practical problem situations in which the consultants took the roles of disturbed people, complainants, and bystanders. The problem situations were ordered so that the initial problems could serve to disconfirm the stereotype that the mentally disturbed are dangerous, with subsequent problems making the probability of dangerousness more ambiguous, as well as to illustrate other points about problems of mental health. In the latter problem situations, the actual occurrence of difficult or dangerous behavior was role-played so as to be contingent on the police cadet's behavior in handling the situation.[13]

Four practical problems were presented. Each problem was handled by a cadet who was given only the advance information which he would probably receive by radio dispatch. After enacting the situation, a critique and discussion was held in which the cadets asked additional questions and we emphasized salient points illustrated by the problem. Then the problem situation was re-enacted with a different cadet. Naturally, the second presentation was handled more effectively, and we felt it was important to give the cadets some experience of success in such situations. Police instructors made valuable contributions to the discussions by clarifying legal and procedural points, and relating illustrative examples from their own experiences. At the same time, they learned some things along with the cadets which they had not known before.

The premise of the first problem was that a depressed person

---

[13] In reality, the probability of danger in any behavioral situation is contingent on many factors, not all of which can be controlled by the police officer. Our purpose here was to reinforce procedures which would minimize the officer's contributing to potential danger unwittingly and also enhance his potential as a helping agent.

sitting near the river was ruminating about his misfortunes, had thought about suicide, but was not considering it seriously. The subject displayed retardation of thinking and emotional reactions, was difficult to engage in conversation, but was responsive to suggestion and amenable to help. As it was acted out, the problem proved to be a good vehicle for sensitizing the police cadets to the possible effects of their own behavior, since the subject was initially passive and uncommunicative. The cadets were forced to try a number of alternative verbal approaches to engage the subject, and to assess their effects by the subject's response. One aspect which came up repeatedly was the policeman's posture and bodily communication. Several cadets stood over the subject, who was seated, with their hands on their hips, the right hand resting just above their holstered service revolver. When this was brought to their attention, they expressed uncertainty about what to do with their hands and the fact that the protruding revolver made placement of their hands awkward when standing. Sitting beside the subject or squatting in front of him relieved this problem and communicated a more helpful attitude.

The second problem involved more elaborate arrangements, including a young adult mental retardate who was merely standing in front of a store, playing with a penny, the complaining storeowner who claimed that the subject was bothering customers and driving away business, and one or two bystanders who were potential sources for verifying the storeowner's complaint. This situation served to discriminate problems associated with limited intelligence from those of emotional disturbance, to highlight the dynamics of the complainant-subject relationship and direct the cadet's attention to mediating the psychological situation rather than merely taking action with the subject of the complaint. The problem served to bring out several misunderstandings. Some cadets assumed that they were obligated to take the retarded person into custody without pursuing other alternatives, such as assessing his level of social skills, his orientation, his proximity to home, and his ability to care for his own needs. Others assumed that the subject had escaped from an institution and were unaware that mental retardates could function in the community. Few of them directed their attention to the complainant and the possibility that merely removing the subject might be followed by another complaint in the near future unless the rights of citizens were clarified for the store-owner and it was pointed out to him that the subject was harmless.

The third problem portrayed an individual seated on a bench for would-be bus riders who acted somewhat uncoordinated and disoriented. He was jovial and friendly, but frequently distracted by stimuli not visible to the onlooker. Although the problem was based on the premise that the subject was on a drug *trip,* the situation required distinguishing this condition from drunkenness or psyschosis with hallucinations. In reality, this is sometimes a difficult discrimination for policemen to make on the street, and the problem was designed to present the cadets with a task which required rather thorough examination and careful reflection as to his legal and policy basis for intervention.

The fourth problem situation was based on an angry paranoid person regaling a street-corner gathering with what approximated, but was not, radical rhetoric. Here the cadet was required not only to make a careful assessment of the situation, but the probability of violent reactions by the subject was made contingent on the cadet's approach and handling of the situation. For example, an abrupt, physical approach without warning produced strong resistance, while an openly visible tack in which the cadet attempted to place himself into the subject's frame of reference and allowed the subject enough psychological distance and advance warning of his planned action that the subject had an opportunity to choose to comply with the officer's request was met with cooperation.[14] Following the problem, the desired approach tactics and the reasons for them were explained to the cadets.

In line with the theory outlined in Chapter III it was expected that experience with these problem situations would loosen the association between mental health problems and dangerousness. The next step was intended to further extinguish that association. The cadets were taken on tours of the Community Mental Health/Mental Retardation Center and the state hospital, in order to familiarize them with each agency's personnel and policies, and

---

[14] See footnote number 13.

to expose them to people with mental health problems under non-threatening conditions.

In addition to learning the physical location of the Mental Health Center, the cadets met with personnel of the center who explained their procedures in handling crisis cases and how the cadets could refer people to them for help. The cadets were advised of the facts that many people whose relatives might want to commit them to an institution could be helped on an outpatient basis, and that the Mental Health Center was trying to screen commitment requests in order to reduce the need for hospitalization. The discussion which followed usually involved the relationship between the center's policies and the various legal and procedural requirements of the police department.

At the state hospital, the cadets toured the county unit, the adolescent unit and the Alcoholic Rehabilitation Unit, met some of the patients and again discussed policies and procedures with the hospital staff.

At a later date, the police cadets met with representatives of a number of community agencies concerned with mental health problems in the Mental Health Association Workshop. Some of the personnel the cadets had met during their tours were among those present. The format of these meetings was to have the agency professionals act as resource people in a day-long series of problem-centered small group discussions led by the consultants. Problems were discussed under four topics: family disturbances, alcoholism, minority group relations, and youth problems.

The tours and the workshop helped to meet the needs for better acquaintance with community resources and referral practices. It was felt that personal acquaintances with other agency personnel would make this information more salient, and that the policemen would feel more confident in making referrals on the basis of this experience.

Family Disturbances

In addition to the information gained during the familiarization phase of the project, we were fortunate to have the benefit of data collected in several background studies of police work by students in the Criminal Justice Project of the University of Texas School of Law.[15] One of these studies dealt with family disturbances.

Bailey (1970) collected data from police records and personally observed 70 incidents of police responses to family disturbances. He also observed training procedures and interviewed both patrolmen and supervisors on their attitudes toward family disturbance situations. In the incidents reviewed by Bailey, there were only three arrests made, two of which involved public drunkenness, and the other, public fighting. There were no public injuries or deaths during the period of the study, nor during the consultation project, despite the fact that national statistics indicate that family disturbances are among the most dangerous situations in which police may become involved.

The low incidence of arrests follows from a deliberate policy of the department of minimal involvement and non-arrest, which is reflected in the cadet training mentioned previously. The policy is based on a philosophy of respect for the individual's dignity in his own home, the rather strong legal sanctions against police action in a private dwelling and the recognition that minimal police involvement in an already tense situation reduces the dangers involved to the policemen. Policemen are instructed that they should not make an arrest except in cases of emergency where there is danger that someone may be physically harmed, and Bailey's data testify to adherence to this policy.

The officers interviewed by Bailey expressed three goals in intervening in family disputes. Listed in order of reported importance, they are maintaining peace and order, maintaining personal safety and providing help to people in trouble. The officers reported seeing the family dispute as an opportunity to practice public relations in line with the department's philosophy that persons who call for police assistance should have a uniformed officer respond to their request. They felt it was important that while explaining to the parties involved the limitations of the policeman's role, and doing what they could within those limitations to restore order, that they also help the subjects involved to avoid embarrassment.

---

[15] Directed by Professor Michael Rosenthal, whose interest in and cooperation with the project is gratefully acknowledged.

Bailey reported that the most frequently observed techniques were advising the complainant that the officer couldn't intervene and advising the complainant of the option of filing a formal complaint. Other techniques observed infrequently were referral to a judge or legal clinic, advising a complainant who wishes to file charges that a cross-complaint may be filed, advising separation of the parties, mediation, and threat of arrest. In line with the policy of minimal intervention and the goals of restoring immediate peace and order, each of these techniques was aimed at a short-range restoration of equilibrium, and the policemen neither voiced nor displayed a commitment to relatively long-term solutions. While the policemen does not see his role nor his abilities as either requiring or allowing him to take on commitments to more permanent resolutions, Bailey noted that the policemen could contribute to beginning such processes if they had and utilized more information on referrals to social and mental health agencies who did have such commitments, and if they received more training in mediation techniques.

There were no referrals to mental health agencies in the cases Bailey observed, but referral to legal sources was present in at least some instances. Therefore, it seemed reasonable that referral itself should not be an obstacle, and that information about referral sources and an emphasis on making it a practice would allow the policeman to make a further contribution in handling family disturbances with minimal conflict in his existing patterns of operation. Training in mediation techniques, however, seemed to present more of a potential for such conflict.

Our efforts at training in this area consisted of making contributions within the existing training program concerning family disturbances, and additional input to both cadet training and the department as a whole in the form of referral information. We participated as observers and discussants in the practical problem training situations concerned with family disturbances and one of the problem-oriented discussion topics in the Mental Health Association Workshop was family disturbances.

However, since both departmental policy and the policemen's self-image emphasized short-term intervention in such incidents, we felt that our most effective contribution would be in providing additional referral information and encouraging its use. Three by five inch cards were prepared which contained the names, addresses and telephone numbers of community agencies arranged in five categories: children and adolescents, disturbed persons, family disturbances, alcoholism, and personal and financial aid. These cards were distributed and explained to the policemen during an assembly period prior to each shift. It was anticipated that this information would also be helpful in dealing with the problems relevant to the additional categories listed, and would provide a tangible follow-up to our training of cadets in handing mental health problems.

Consideration of teaching policemen to mediate family conflicts involves a number of issues which can be fruitfully explored. First it might be noted that the departmental policy differs in both kind and specificity in relation to family disturbances and mentally disturbed behavior. While both categories are viewed as potentially dangerous by policemen, the character of the danger ascribed to each is somewhat different. In the case of family disturbances, one rationale for limiting intervention is the potential danger to the officer. For mentally disturbed persons, the rationale for intervention, both legally and procedurally is the individual's potential danger to himself or others, but not specifically to the officer. Thus, two categories of behavior in which most mental health professionals would assume a high degree of overlap are separated artificially by institutionalized distinctions.

The practical effect of this distinction is that policemen tend to regard behavior in a family disturbance as *normal* for that setting, while the same behavior in a different setting would be considered *disturbed* and possibly grounds for intervention. This is not to say that the policeman might not consider the family in which disturbed behavior occurs to be *disturbed,* but rather to emphasize that the public or private nature of the setting in which the behavior occurs influences the perception and interpretation of behavior occurring in those settings and in turn influences the kinds of decision rules which are invoked. Perhaps it is easier for the policeman to observe the situational pressures leading to disturbed behavior in the family setting than in the public display of disturbed behavior by the isolated individual, with the result that it is less necessary to classify that behavior as *abnormal* in order to comprehend it.

In any case, these distinctions limit the policeman's readiness to define the behavior he observes in family disturbances as relevant to mental health intervention and may constrain the alternative goals he might consider appropriate to achieve through attempts at mediation.

On the other hand, from the standpoint of community mental health ideology, there is a definite plus to be considered from not applying the label *abnormal* to an increasing array of behaviors, but rather to learn to understand behavior from the standpoint of the situation and the individual's background, and attempt to deal with it in terms of that understanding. Accordingly, our approach to training in handling family disturbances was to attempt to reduce the conflict for the policeman at the level of action taken rather than at the level of defining behavior. We pointed out that mental health and social agencies could be helpful for problems which would not fall within the boundaries of behavior covered by the *lunacy* ordinance, and that one did not have to be *crazy* to take advantage of such help. Our expectations were that giving the police cadets an acceptable alternative to nonintervention would increase their confidence in handling such situations without requiring significantly more involvement than was consistent with departmental policy. Because of the policy constraints and in keeping with the assumptions of supervisors that the policeman would learn more sophisticated techniques for handling family disturbances as he became more experienced, we decided to limit our efforts to develop more complex techniques for mediating of family disturbances to consultation activities with individual officers around specific problem cases until such time as we could demonstrate a sufficient problem basis for offering such training to groups of policemen.

Chapter VI

COMMUNITY AGENCY CONFERENCE

The meetings are useful because the people concerned are all involved in public service work. Though we work in different areas of community services, the people with whom we work have problems which cannot be confined to any one agency's area of responsibility. It follows then that the members of the different agencies cannot be effective unless the problems of our clientele are treated as a whole rather than in segments.

—Quotation from a police officer's evaluation of the interagency meetings.

THE IDEA OF A SERIES of meetings between police personnel and workers from mental health-related agencies in the community was first suggested in the original planning of the project by policemen who expressed a need for bringing additional resources to bear on problems of disturbed behavior. As the project progressed, this concept took on additional meanings in the form of providing for policemen more referral information and alternative ways of looking at disturbed behavior, for workers from other agencies first-hand acquaintance with policemen and an understanding of their functions and constraints, and for all better relationships among community resources which could result in improved help-giving services to the people of the community.

In the beginning it is possible that the concept of the meetings implied for some policemen that other agencies should assume responsibility for mental health problems and relieve the police of an unwanted burden. As it developed, however, any such unrealistic expectations were overcome by an appreciation of mutual involvement and responsibility which led to cooperative planning.

81

Community Organization Concepts

The plan of the meetings, which were called the Community Agency Conference, followed an organizational strategy described by Rhodes, *et al.* (1968) for developing community agency organization in a multi-problem neighborhood. Key community agencies were identified whose activities were concerned with some phase of mental health problems and whose workers and clients had, or potentially could have, some interaction with policemen as part of the problem with which the agency was concerned. Each consultant was assigned to make contact with two of these agencies and explore their interest in participating in the Community Agency Conference.

Our first step was to contact the chief administrator of each agency, explain the concept of the conference, and invite nomination of personnel to represent the agency at the meetings. Many of these agencies had already participated in the Mental Health Association workshops and had at least some agenda which interested them in the conference. We asked specifically for front-line worker representatives since we wanted to affect this level of activity in the community. From previous experience, the author believed that personnel at the front-line level were more free to engage in problem-solving exchanges with similar workers from other agencies and would be less constrained by concerns about *territoriality* and public image. At the same time, most agencies were already involved at the administrative level in interagency planning through the Community Council and their involvement at the administrative level in these meetings might represent a duplication of effort. Rather than competing with these efforts, the conference was seen as a means of extending the basis for cooperation to different levels of organization.

Police personnel selected to attend the meetings included the officers who were assigned duty as Captain of Police, supervisory personnel from the Homicide, Vice, and Crime Prevention details of the Criminal Investigation Division, and representative supervisors from the Uniformed Division. The Captain of Police position has a key function in the day-to-day operation of the department in that he coordinates the activity of the department during a shift, approving or disapproving arrests for bookings and other dispositions, including suggesting alternative dispositions such as referrals to mental health or other agencies. The Homicide, Vice, and Crime Prevention details are responsible for cases involving mental health problems, drugs, and juveniles, respectively.

The consultants then proceeded to establish relationships with the agency representatives and act as a liaison between the agency and the police department. Occasionally they were called upon in a consultative capacity by the agency workers to deal with problems of an interagency nature or within that particular agency itself. These relationships helped the consultants to introduce issues in the meetings which might not have been presented otherwise, and to follow-up specific problems which were raised in the meetings with the relevant agencies.

Another concern was the question of turf, and the effect on spontaneity and openness of being a guest or a host in a particular setting. We decided to rotate the meeting places among the agencies, so as to dilute this concern and to provide exposure to and increased familiarity with each agency's facilities. Within this framework, we gave priority to meeting places which were visited infrequently by other agency personnel and with which they were least likely to be familiar. Each meeting was preceded by a tour of the facility and a brief description of program by the host agency representatives. This necessarily tended to focus the discussion on problems associated with that particular setting, and the role of the consultants was to attempt to focus the attention of the group on the dimensions of the problems which were of mutual concern.

We expected that these meetings would have effects beyond the specific personnel attending them in that each representative would probably discuss the meetings formally or informally with other workers in his or her agency, might introduce information or attitudes resulting from these meetings into intraagency problem solving, and might promote personal contacts between other agency personnel as appropriate problems arose. Accordingly, we predicted a diffusion effect which should influence the attitudes of the agency as a whole as a result of these meetings, as well as changes in specific cooperative practices.

The Interagency Meetings

The meetings were held once each month from 12:00 noon to 2:00 PM. After a tour of the facility, lunch was either provided by the agency or brought in, and discussions proceeded. In all, seven meetings were held during the period of the project. A list of the agencies participating in these meetings is presented in Appendix I. A summary of each meeting was prepared and distributed to each participant prior to the next meeting.

A Content Analysis

Although problems discussed at the meetings tended to be influenced by the setting, there were some persistent concerns which recurred in all meetings. Diagnostically, it can be assumed that such recurrent themes are symptoms of problems which the help-giving services are having difficulty resolving. The problem topics arising most often were drug abuse including alcoholism; psychiatric emergencies, including suicides and commitment procedures; hospital escapees; juvenile runaways; and the fringe community attracted by the presence of the university, the so-called *street people*.

At the level of procedures, topics arose in a more systematically phasic manner, which may be some indication that the participants were achieving a sense of closure on these concerns. The initial meetings were heavily concerned with discussions about referral information and processes, and interagency information sharing. These gradually gave way to concerns with coordinating new programs and services which were being developed. Prominent among these was a new 24-hour telephone crisis service, which was seen as potentially meeting some of the needs for coordinating services after the 5:00 PM closing hour of most agencies, and plans for new services in alcoholic detoxification and drug treatment programs. The conference served as a convenient vehicle for developing, coordinating, and publicizing these new projects. In turn, these issues gave rise to an increasing focus on the functions of the conference itself, and how it might serve to develop policy guidelines and effect the coordination of procedures and services.

In looking at the problems which persisted in the attention of the conference participants, it is worth raising the question of what common elements these problems contain in an effort to understand better the limitations of the network of human services as a community coping mechanism. Each of these problem areas has an acute demand characteristic when viewed as a stimulus for community reaction. They represent threats to some of the central norms and values upon which the community organization is founded: individual responsibility, the integrity of the family, respect for authority, and, indeed, the preservation of life.

However, several other problems also present these kinds of challenges, such as criminal behavior which is not defined as relevant for mental health or social service intervention, and the various autoplastic psychological reactions which may impair the functioning of the individual but do not visibly effect the functioning of the community system. The difference, then, seems to lie in the fact that these latter forms of behavior fall more or less wholly within the purview of a single major behavior mediating institution of the community where there is relatively broad consensus as to the diagnosis of the problem for society and the appropriate intervention, leaving aside for the moment considerations of the validity of this perception and its effectiveness for community life in the long run; while the problems which commanded the continuing attention of the conference are those about which the community has not reached consensus as to diagnosis or intervention. These problems are defined and prescribed for differently in the legal, mental health and social systems, with resolutions coming only idiosyncratically in the individual case, and even then probably somewhat arbitrarily and haphazardly. In addition, these problems share a characteristic which is analogous to what Goffman (1969) refers to as "the insanity of place"; that is, they represent a rupture of relationships and the associated expectations which are assumed to apply to members of the community social system, and unlike the *clearly criminal* or the *clearly sick,* there is no established role, even among those deviant roles which society tolerates, through which the community can relate to such persons consistently.

Thus, the apparent paradox of the conference being able to alleviate some of its concerns with procedures while at the same

time achieving little reduction in its concerns for certain problems
may perhaps be understood from the perspective that such a resolution lies outside of the purview of the network of services as it
functions presently. According to this view, it is expectable that
the conference would begin to become concerned with its own
functions. How this came about deserves further analysis from
the standpoint of the process of the conference as a group.

A Process Analysis

The initial meeting began with mutual introductions and was
marked by a degree of formality and constraint. While many of
the participants were acquainted with each other, they were not
accustomed to interacting in a setting in which they were also
being observed by others with whom they were unfamiliar. Thus,
a period of testing and observation was necessary. However, as the
participants demonstrated their mutual concerns with problems
and began to exchange information, the discussions became more
spontaneous and relaxed.

Viewed from another perspective, each participant had certain
agenda items which they needed to unload. This process was described by some participants as *griping and ventilating*. If this had
been the primary motivation for participation, however, then it
would be expected that the unloading stage would be followed
by a termination of the meeting. Instead, once this process was
completed, the conference participants began to explore ways in
which they could become a group in themselves by focusing on
the functions which the conference could perform. Here, the
participants had to assess seriously their investment in the format,
and their freedom and willingness to participate in what was for
them a new social form, a superordinate vehicle for attempting to
solve problems.

The change in focus was marked by the introduction of discussion to the effect that certain problem areas suffered from a
lack of explicit interagency policies and guidelines, by suggestions
that participants might form subcommittees to study and formu-
late guidelines, and by proposals that the conference serve officially as a liaison for interagency problems. This is a critical phase
in the formation of such a group, for a latent issue in these pro-

posals is the degree and source of power which such a group could or should have. Among the considerations in making this additional commitment are the freedom and willingness of the participants to share their influence potential through cooperative actions, and their perception of the effects of such a commitment on their standing in their own agency. In addition, there is the question of the subjective estimates of the costs of involvement, which are immediate, versus the benefits, which are more remote. In general, this stage represents a shift from attendance to participation.

Once this step is completed, it is to be expected that the members of the conference will begin to influence each other's attitudes towards community problems, as distinguished from merely increasing information about community services. Since this is a mutual process, it is expected that the attitudes of the participants will show increasing convergence. Along with this convergence in attitudes there should also be an increase in interagency transactions outside of the meetings to deal with specific problems.

For this group, the shift to participation occurred after the third meeting and was marked by an increase in subgroup meetings concerned with such problems as coordinating follow-up action on suicide attempts, the legal status of persons participating in drug treatment programs, and the clarification of procedures for handling runaway juveniles. Data on changes in attitudes toward community problems are reported in the section on evaluation.

The effects observed as a result of the conference should be regarded only as indicating a potential for improved human services in the community. To suggest that the conference had fulfilled its purpose during the seven meetings would be overstating the case. Realistically, the participants can only begin to come to agreement about community problems and act toward them out of a consensual attitudinal framework to the extent that they, as frontline workers, have some degrees of freedom to make decisions about particular cases or classes of problems within the community's definition of and reactions toward such problems. In a larger sense, the community's stance toward many human problems remains conflicted, and the conference is not a sufficient vehicle for resolving that conflict. However, the conference has demonstrated that within the latitude available, there is sufficient room for improving cooperation and coordinating services to make such a project worthwhile.

Toward the end of the conference series, the question of whether the meetings should be continued in the future arose because of the complications of scheduling the meetings during the summer vacation period. In order to assess the feelings of the participants towards continuation, a questionnaire was distributed to the participants, asking them to answer four questions:

1. Do you feel the meetings have been worthwhile?
2. Please describe in what ways the meetings have or have not been useful.
3. Do you feel the meetings should be continued? Why?
4. If further meetings are held, how could they be improved?

Participants were asked to indicate their agency affiliation on the form, but not to sign their names. Since there was more than one representative from each agency, some measure of confidentiality of responses was possible.

Out of fourteen questionnaires, eleven were returned completed. In response to item one, ten persons indicated the meetings had been worthwhile and one said that some of them had been so. The ways in which the meetings were useful reported in item two were open ended, but can be summarized under four categories, with the number of responses indicated for each category:

Meeting and getting to know other agency personnel: five.

Developing better communications and relationships with specific people in other agencies: two.

Understanding the problems and procedures of other agencies, correcting misunderstandings, and improving coordination: eight.

Better understanding the overall pattern of service functions: two.

Under item three, nine persons indicated that they thought the meetings should continue, one responded to this item with a question mark, and one felt that the meetings had served their purpose and should be discontinued. Reasons for continuation given by those favoring continuation included six persons who cited the usefulness of the meetings indicated under item two and the fact that there was much more work to be done, and one who said the meetings were the only systematic form of communication between agencies which existed to his knowledge. Two persons gave no specific reasons for continuation. A representative of the Community Mental Health Center reported noticing a definite change toward more understanding and acceptance of mental health problems by police officers, and improvement in the representative's own appreciation of the problems which police officers face.

Suggested improvements mentioned under item four were very consistent in focusing on continued efforts to structure the meetings toward developing policies in relation to particular problems. It was suggested that the effects of possible guidelines on particular agencies should be discussed openly, that the representatives should discuss the proceedings of the conference with other workers in their agencies, and that they should report back to the conference on specific changes which their agencies were making in response to the deliberations of the conference.

The results of the questionnaire support the contention that the Community Agency Conference is a useful form to achieve interagency cooperation, and indicate the commitment of the participants to developing coordinated community services. This promising beginning deserves continued support and development.

PART III

EVALUATION

INTRODUCTION

E VALUATION OF A PROJECT implies something more than mere measurement. In this section, an attempt is made to present various kinds of evidence bearing on the effects of the consultation relationship, and to relate that evidence to the goals of the project so as to draw some conclusions about what the project may mean to the Police Department and to the community in the future.

Some kinds of data could not be collected, and some goals conceived as eventual effects of the project were not expected to be reached during the demonstration period. External conditions which might have affected the results on some measures could not always be controlled, so that the process of inferring changes as a result of the project could not always be made unambiguous. Within these limitations, however, it is possible to assess the accomplishment of some immediate goals of the project and to measure progress which may be instrumental in the eventual attainment of other goals. Finally, some observations on the problems of evaluative research can be made from the opportunities and barriers to assessment which arose during the project, but which could not be incorporated in the design of this evaluation.

The goals to be assessed encompass different conceptual levels and necessarily involve sampling from different domains. Initial concern must focus on the more proximal intermediate goals and the indications of progress towards more distant objectives. Thus, one area to be assessed is the evaluation given the project by members of the Police Department, evidence for the survival and continuation of this form of activity beyond the demonstration period, and specific changes visible to the policemen themselves. This evidence is reviewed in Chapter VII.

A second domain consists of evidence for accomplishment of goals pertinent to secondary prevention in the form of early identification and treatment. Within the purview of police activity, this evidence comes from changes in referrals for mental health services, and from changes in the handling of mental health crises. The data are more directly behavioral and can be treated statistically. Chapter VIII contains the results which are pertinent to this question.

A third focus is evidence for attitude changes which may affect more broadly the policemen's reactions to disturbed or disturbing behavior, his relationships with other agencies, and his feelings about the community and its problems. From this data it is possible not only to assess some of the effects of this project, but to speculate on possible alternatives for future activities. Examination of these concerns is the content of Chapter IX.

VIABILITY OF THE CONSULTATION PROGRAM

T HE BEST CONCEIVED and most effective programs will not survive long unless they are well received by those whom they effect. The historical path of program innovation is littered with the casualties of demonstration programs which were technically correct but which failed to capture, and sometimes failed to seek, the cooperation and support of the potential recipients. An effort was made to overcome this problem in the police consultation project by involving policemen in the planning of the project at the outset, and seeking their advice and opinions in periodic reviews of progress. No matter what the statistical data show, a discarded demonstration project is in some respects a social failure. Therefore, it is appropriate to examine the effects of this project from the viewpoint of the Police Department.

Although some of this evidence is in the form of testimonial reports, which are subject to halo effects and not necessarily based on actual behavioral changes, it constitutes an important source of data for evaluating projects of this type. Favorable testimonials reflect the degree of commitment and involvement, enthusiasm if you will, which the project has generated, and this variable is both critical for program survival and a potential contributor to its effectiveness. A program which can generate support and a sense of involvement from its recipients is likely to benefit from the efforts of those thus affected to see that it does succeed. In addition, it is possible to support this testimonial evidence with indications of behavioral and organizational changes related to the testimonial reports.

Continuation of the Project

An important question, then, is the survival and continuation of the project. At the time of this writing, some six months after the expiration of the demonstration period, the consultation program is not only continuing but expanding its involvement, particularly in the area of training. Equally important, the program has also survived the termination of the author's association with it and is being conducted currently by a colleague who formerly served as one of the student consultants.[16] Thus, it may be inferred that the program is seen as valuable in its own right by the Police Department.

The activities conducted as part of the project have received enthusiastic support within the department, and, while details have not been finalized as yet, financial support of the program from public sources has been promised. Activities which have been expanded include more time and emphasis on training in practical problem situations for police cadets and an increase in the range of topics covered. Police cadets now receive orientation visits to several different community agencies in addition to those included originally and specific time has been included in the training program to cover referral sources and processes. Plans are underway to conduct special programs in drug education, suicide intervention, mental retardation, and cooperative relationships between law enforcement officials and school personnel. The possibility of a research study on the selection of police candidates is being explored currently as a result of discussions of this topic with administrators during the project.

The Police Department's Evaluation

Police Chief Robert Miles asked members of his staff to submit evaluations of the project, which were collated and condensed in a letter to the author. With his permission, this report is reproduced here.

> Since this program involved a number of related projects I shall endeavor to comment separately on each of these phases.
> PARTICIPATION OF GRADUATE PSYCHOLOGY STUDENTS: The active participation of these students with the police in personally witnessing the problems encountered in the performance of their duties materially enhanced the effectiveness of these students in their consulting

---

[16] David Hopkinson, Ph.D.

activities. This knowledge should also prove invaluable to them in the future in other fields.

COMMUNITY AGENCY CONFERENCES: Representatives from eight local agencies met monthly with members of our Criminal Investigation Division Detail who are assigned to investigate offenses against the person. This phase of the program, I feel, was mutually profitable to members of these agencies as well as our officers in developing a better understanding of each other's problems and arriving at procedures which would make our efforts more productive. As a result, my officers are now in a much better position to provide assistance to disturbed, aged, or deprived people through appropriate agencies.

The inauguration of the *Hot Line*[17] service to disturbed persons and the relationship that has been established with my department has enabled us to make many new contacts and to be of material assistance to the persons involved.

INSERVICE TRAINING: The regular college course in psychology as it relates to mentally disturbed people, as conducted by Dr. Mann, has proved quite valuable to our officers who enrolled. Dr. Mann's familiarity with police officers and their daily tasks contributed much to the success of this course of training. Conversely, his discussions with our officers on these topics at that time added to the effectiveness of his subsequent consultation project with all of our officers.

LISTING OF REFERRAL SOURCES: The laminated pocket size card distributed to all officers listing the major sources with their addresses and telephone numbers has proven quite valuable. In fact, one hour's discussion of this subject is now included in the regular training program for all new officers.

Cadet Training

PROJECT UNDERSTANDING: This participation of the student consultants as moderators in each of the group discussions with representative teenagers, adults and our cadets has made this an outstandingly effective phase of our training of new officers.

STRESS TRAINING: Three training films and a training manual were purchased with funds from this project. This project has proved to be unusually successful and it is planned to continue to include it as a regular part of the training program for all new officers.

PRACTICAL PROBLEMS IN HUMAN RELATIONS: This program covering role playing by the psychology students in simulated situations of mental and emotional disturbances has been very effective in preparing these officers when they are confronted with similar situations in the field.

---

[17] A 24-hour crisis-oriented telephone service.

TOURS OF INSTITUTIONS FOR THE MENTALLY DISTURBED: This has provided the cadets with firsthand knowledge of the facilities available as well as an opportunity to make personal contact with some of these patients.

I have endeavored to set forth above a general evaluation of the various phases of this program. As I believe we agreed at the outset of the project, however, it would be almost impossible to refer to any specific, tangible evidence of its effectiveness. I can definitely state, however, that there has been a significant increase in the number of referrals we have made to the interested agencies. Further, through a mutual understanding of our respective problems and operations a much better climate has developed in our contacts with each other.

Certainly, many of my officers, particularly those just entering police work, have developed a much higher degree of expertise in handling the emotionally disturbed and in counseling with them.

You may be assured that Dr. Hopkinson is working closely with us and I have every intention of continuing the program in every manner possible.

Additional Indications

At another level, the popularity of a program such as this and the enthusiasm of the policemen for it can be inferred indirectly from the reactions of other police officers who are not members of the Police Department which is directly involved. As it happens, both the campus police force of the University of Texas, and the headquarters of the state police; the Department of Public Safety, are located in Austin. In addition to their police activities, both of these organizations conduct the training activities for their respective systems throughout the state. Because of their proximity to each other and their periodic cooperation in cases of mutual jurisdiction, members of all three of these police organizations are well acquainted with each other. Requests have been received from both the University of Texas Police and the Department of Public Safety to conduct similar training programs for their organizations.

Since the author was not personally acquainted with any members of either of these organizations prior to the requests, and since the project received no news media publicity, their knowledge of and interest in the project would have had to come from their interactions with members of the Austin Police Department. It can be assumed that the policemen involved in these contacts gave favorable reports of the activity of the program. While this evidence is also a kind of testimonial, it stems from a more private level of discourse. As such, it tends to justify the assumption that the enthusiastic approval of the program reported by members of the police department reflects their genuine feelings and is not merely public *window dressing*.

Another indication of the effects of the program is an important policy change in the department which resulted directly from the interactions of the Community Agency Conference. Because of agreements made through the conference between policemen and representatives of a volunteer organization which offers services to persons with drug problems, policemen who encounter persons experiencing *bad trips* from drugs are now directed to contact a member of the medical staff of the service and turn such persons over to them for care, whereas previously such persons were placed in jail. This policy change provides the policemen with a meaningful and appropriate alternative in such cases and improves the probability of such persons receiving appropriate care and treatment. Not incidentally, it also sets an important precedent for cooperative agreements with other community agencies in handling problems of mutual concern.

Finally, an unplanned observation provides an additional bit of behavioral evidence for the effects of the program. Recently, the author happened to be in Austin on other business and stopped in to visit the Police Department. While the author was chatting informally with the officer in charge of the Homicide detail, a patrolman entered the office. The patrolman had brought a young man to the department because he thought the man might be in need of immediate help. The officer reported that while he was investigating a traffic accident, the young man approached him, obviously distressed, and asked insistently if he could sit in his police car. Inside the car, the man told the policeman that he was a homosexual and that he had a problem of exposing himself to people. He said he would feel better if he could just sit in the car for a while. The patrolman offered to assist the man in getting help for his problem, and the man agreed to accompany him to the police station.

At the request of the officer in charge of the Homicide Detail, the author agreed to interview the man to see what might be done for him. The man reported that he had been in psychotherapy for a brief time, and that he had begun to gain some understanding of his problem. However, he had recently been under increased stress and had encountered a series of disappointments. His therapist was out of town at the time, and while on his way downtown to shop he saw the police officer and was seized with the impulse to expose himself to the policeman. However, he said that the policeman was so kind and understanding that he "could not do that (expose himself) to him." After some additional inquiry, the man indicated that he had now had an opportunity to regain his composure, did not feel the need of additional help, and was confident that he could control himself. The author was satisfied that this was the case, and advised the man to contact his psychotherapist's agency if he should experience additional difficulty. The author explained this opinion to the patrolman and complimented him on his actions. The patrolman then drove the man downtown so that he could do his shopping.

To the clinician, the case presents a rich opportunity to examine the multiple unarticulated needs and goals which the man's behavior would appear to be serving, but it is clear that the policeman involved saw this case as a challenge of a human being in need. Apart from the stereotype of the attitudes which policemen are supposed to hold toward sexual deviancy, and this case negates that stereotype, situations of this type would present a value and attitude conflict to most ordinary citizens. The fact that the officer was able to ignore the social stigma attached to the sexual deviations which the man attributed to himself, and to address himself to the human needs which the man was expressing in such a way that the man was helped to regain his composure is both remarkable and laudatory.

Critical incidents such as this one lend substance to the evaluation of social interventions. They amplify dramatically effects which may not, and sometimes cannot be obtained through statistical analysis, and exemplify for others involved in such programs the goals which the organization is trying to accomplish. Of course, they must be balanced against the occurrence of negatively valued incidents, which may not be as visible, in order to justify their status as evidence of positive changes. Still, they are the kind of data which most people, including policemen, use and can relate to in evaluating their own performances. They deserve a place in the evaluative process.

In summary, the data reported here indicate that the activities of the consultation project have succeeeded in demonstrating their usefulness to the Police Department, the program has continued and expanded beyond the original demonstration period, and there is every reason to expect that the activities will survive as a regular part of the police organization's functioning. Some tentative evidence on changes effected by the project has been presented, and in the next two chapters the kinds of changes which have occurred are considered in more detail.

Chapter VIII

CHANGES IN CRISIS MANAGEMENT

THROUGHOUT THE PLANNING and conduct of the project one of the main goals has been to effect a change in the way policemen manage crisis situations involving human behavior. Within the framework of preventive terminology which community mental health has borrowed from public health, such interventions can be conceived of as having either primary or secondary preventive impact in reducing psychosocial disability. For instance, Caplan (1964) describes a strategy of primary prevention through intervention into normal life crises in such a way that the resolution of the crisis results in healthy growth. Logically, primary preventive intervention must precede the development of seriously maladaptive behavior patterns. Once such patterns have developed, it is still possible to intervene in a preventive sense, but in this latter case the goal is to use the crisis situation as a ripe opportunity for change which can mitigate the maladaptive pattern, thus reducing the probability of occurrence of more serious, chronic difficulties. This latter practice is a secondary preventive strategy.

In general, interventions which involve the use of treatment or services for an existing maladaptive behavior problem are classified as secondary prevention. Many of the cases which policemen encounter in responding to crisis situations are of this nature. For example, the large majority of family disputes to which policemen are called have a previous history of interpersonal difficulties which cannot be expected to be resolved without fairly extensive treatment intervention. Persons who have attempted suicide will automatically come under the province of secondary prevention. However, the distinction between these two types of prevention is not always easy to make in some cases. Secondary preventive efforts

102

may occasionally have primary preventive effects, as when successful early intervention in an adult family problem results in an improved home situation for the growth and development of children, or when the relatives and friends of a person who has attempted suicide are helped to manage their emotional reactions to the event. There are other opportunities for more direct primary preventive interventions in police work which will be discussed later. The events to be considered here can be thought of generally as having secondary prevention as their aim.

Family Disturbances

As discussed earlier, the brunt of training which police cadets receive for intervening in family disputes directs them to minimize their involvement in such affairs. The reasoning behind this is that family disturbances are potentially dangerous situations which at the same time, because of the emotionally charged atmosphere, contain strong incentives for becoming involved. It is thought that training the novice policeman towards an attitude of noninvolvement until he gains more experience will help to protect him. The consultation strategy was to provide the policeman with ways of intervening which would maintain a degree of protection while allowing him to interject some potentially helpful information into the situation. This was done by making information about referral sources readily available, providing encouragement and training in its use, as well as specific training in crisis intervention.

As an outcome of this strategy, it is to be expected that policemen should then increase the frequency with which they took some action in family disturbances, in the form of providing referral information and personal or social advice, as opposed to taking no action and relying on a disclaimer of no lawful jurisdiction, or providing legally-oriented advice, such as telling the parties that they can file charges.

METHOD: To test this expectation, police records of family disturbance were reviewed and analyzed. This process presented numerous difficulties which were not anticipated and limited the information which could be collected. In police records, all disturbance reports are filed together with miscellaneous incidents and complaints, only some of which are actually family disturbances, and the number of such reports is voluminous. In 1969, the department recorded 110,602 miscellaneous incidents. Thus, it was necessary to sample from this pool in order to obtain family disturbance reports. Moreover, since these incidents are seldom, if ever, of any subsequent legal consequence, they consist usually of brief descriptions which contain little of the information about such events that a researcher might desire. Bard and Berkowitz (1967) have also noted the scarcity of information in such records, referring to the family disturbance as an official *nonevent.* They employed a specialized record-keeping system in their project which was not feasible with the number of officers involved in this program.

Accordingly, brief time periods of five days each were selected at random at the beginning and end of the project.[18] All reports of family disturbances recorded during these periods were copied and analyzed. This procedure yielded a before and after design, with the records of the *before* period serving as a control group. The information available permitted only two kinds of classifications which were meaningful for purposes of this evaluation. Reports were coded as to whether or not any action was taken by the officer. Giving advice, providing protection, or making a referral were classified as *action taken.* Declining to intervene, informing of the possibility of filing charges, and reports in which no action was reported or necessary, as when the complainants denied a dispute or had settled the issue before the officer's arrival, were classified as *no action.* Those reports which were classified as *action taken* were coded further according to whether the intervention consisted of legal or personal/social action. Thus, referral to a lawyer, custody arrest, and the use of the policeman's presence to force compliance with a legal order were considered legal actions, while personal advice or discussion about settling the dispute, referrals to social agencies, or helping to calm or reassure the participants were recorded as personal/social actions.

---

[18] The magnitude of the task can be estimated from these figures. There would be an average of 303 miscellaneous incident reports per day. For each five-day period there would be 1,515 reports, or a total of 3,030, to be screened.

TABLE I

DISTRIBUTION OF INTERVENTIONS IN FAMILY DISTURBANCES

	Before		Time After		Total
Intervention	f^*	$p^\dagger$	f	p	f
Action taken	6	.40	23	.52	29
No action	9	.60	21	.48	30
Total	15	1.00	44	1.00	59

* Frequency.   † Proportion.

RESULTS: The data obtained from the above procedures were analyzed to determine if the proportion of actions taken in family disputes increased during the project. The distribution of the reports in each category are presented in Table I.

The proportion of cases in which action was taken before and after the project were compared and the probability that the differences obtained were a result of chance was determined by reference to a normal distribution. The Z score for this difference was .92, a score which could be expected to occur by chance 18 percent of the time in different samples. Using the criterion that an obtained difference should have a probability of occurrence by chance less than five percent of the time to be considered significant, the increase in the proportion of cases in which action was taken is not large enough to justify the assumption that similar increases would be found reliably in other time samples.

The distribution of kinds of action within those cases in which action was taken was then analyzed by an identical procedure. The frequency and proportion of cases categorized according to this procedure are presented in Table II.

Comparing the proportion of personal/social interventions in the *after* sample with the proportion of such cases in the *before* sample, the Z score of the difference is 2.06, which would be expected to occur by chance less than two percent of the time. These results indicate a significant change in the kinds of interventions occurring when any action is taken, even though there was not a significant increase in the tendency to take action. Thus, in the face of the early training emphasis on minimum intervention and

TABLE II

DISTRIBUTION OF TYPES OF INTERVENTIONS IN
FAMILY DISTURBANCES

Type of Intervention	Before		After		Total
	f	p	f	p	f
Legal	5	.83	12	.52	17
Personal/social	1	.17	11	.48	12
Total	6	1.00	23	1.00	29

the fact that some of the family disturbance situations do not permit taking any action, these results suggest that the project was successful in changing the kind of interventions which are made in family disturbances.

It may also be noted that the number of family disturbance reports obtained in the second time sample is considerably larger than in the first sample. While this difference may be due to any number of factors, including more diligence in filing reports, it is interesting to note that the increase is approximately of the same order as the increase in family disturbances handled by the Family Crisis Intervention Unit in Bard and Berkowitz's New York project, compared to the number of such cases handled by the control precinct (1970, p. 23).

Suicide Attempts

Another area which affords opportunities for crisis intervention is in the handling of suicide attempts. Here the responsibility for intervention lies more with the medical treatment facilities than with the individual policeman, typically with the hospital emergency room staff. However, both members of the Police Department and the Community Mental Health/Mental Retardation center were concerned about the number of suicide attempts and their management. Studies of the handling of such emergencies have revealed a startlingly small percentage of such cases which receive any psychiatric or other mental health attention; frequently, the practice is to treat the physical condition resulting from the suicide attempt and release the patient. The impression was that this was the case in Austin.

Through the Community Agency Conference, Police and Mental Health Center representatives discussed procedures for insuring better management and follow-up of such cases. Since the public hospital which provided the emergency room service was not represented in the conference, the Mental Health Center arranged to contact the hospital medical staff to discuss the problem.

As a result of these efforts, it was expected that the proportion of suicide attempts taken to the hospital which were subsequently admitted or referred for mental health care would increase at the end of the project over what it was at the beginning.

METHOD: Again, time samples were taken on a *before* and *after* basis. The number of cases was smaller and locating the reports was considerably easier than was the case with the family disturbances. Samples were obtained for one-month periods, with the *before* sample serving as a control group. Once again, the reports were brief but it was possible to obtain information about the method used, potential lethality, and disposition. Dispositions were coded as *treated and released,* or *admitted or referred* (to a mental health resource).

There were no significant differences between the two time samples in the proportions of different methods used, or in the potential lethality of particular methods, such as taking four aspirins as opposed to taking fifty powerful tranquilizers. Thus, any differences obtained can be assumed to reflect changes in intervention practices, rather than severity of the attempt.

RESULTS: The distribution of the two types of dispositions in both time samples are presented in Table III. The increase in the proportion of cases admitted or referred across time is statistically significant. The Z score for the difference between the proportions is 1.88, which would occur by chance only three percent of the time.

These results suggest a significant change in the handling of suicide attempts in the direction of increasing the opportunities for secondary prevention.

Referrals to Mental Health Services

In addition to the data presented above which reflect changes in the referral-making process, it is also possible to assess the effectiveness with which these referrals were made by analyzing

TABLE III

DISTRIBUTION OF THE DISPOSITIONS OF SUICIDE
ATTEMPT CASES

Disposition	Before		Time After		Total
	f	*p*	*f*	*p*	*f*
Treated and released	20	.80	20	.65	40
Admitted or referred	5	.20	11	.35	16
Total	25	1.00	31	1.00	56

changes in the number of persons who followed through on the referral advice and presented themselves for treatment.

METHOD: Beginning in April, 1970, the Community Mental Health/Mental Retardation Center published statistical reports on the number of cases seeking services according to referral sources. It was possible to obtain data from these reports on the number of referrals received from the police and courts at the beginning and end of the project. Since the center was in the process of development, both expanding its services and increasing the knowledge of their availability, it was important to obtain an appropriate control group in order to infer that any increase of police and court referrals was not simply a reflection of an overall increase in either availability or visibility of mental health services. Accordingly, the number of referrals obtained from the public schools, other social service agencies, and other hospital or medical facilities (not including the state mental hospital) were collected as a control group. The average number of referrals from these three sources for each month were compared with those from the police and courts. Since the number of referrals fluctuates from month to month, and this fluctuation cannot be assumed to be independent of the referring agencies, a sample was taken for the first six months for which data were available at the beginning of project (April, 1970, through September, 1970) and compared to a sample of the same six-month period at the end of the project (April, 1971, through September, 1971) so as to control for periodic or seasonal variations. Some training and consultation activities were being conducted during the latter part of the control, or *before* time span. However, it was assumed that the project could not have had a significant effect at that time, and, in any case, the effect would not be to create artificial differences between the time periods sampled. If anything, this sampling procedure would tend to reduce the likelihood of finding significant differences.

RESULTS: The data indicate that there was a statistically significant increase in the number of police/court referrals to the Mental Health Center from beginning to end of the project, while the change in referrals from other sources over this time period was not significant. The number of referrals from the two groups for each time period are presented in Table IV.

From Table IV it can be seen that the number of referrals from each source was practically the same during the *before* time sample, and therefore, the other social agencies provide an appropriate control group. Since referrals were nearly equal for the two sources in the *before* sample, the assumption that the early activities had not effected police referrals seems tenable. The *t* statistic calculated to determine the significance of the difference in police/court referrals between time samples was 4.10, with 5 degrees of freedom, and would be obtained by chance less than one percent of the time, using a two-tailed test. The *t* ratio for the difference in referrals from the other social agencies in the two time samples was .88 which is not statistically significant. It can be concluded that the number of referrals from the police/court source did increase as a result of the project activities. While not all of the re-

TABLE IV

NUMBER OF REFERRALS FROM POLICE/COURT AND OTHER SOCIAL AGENCIES BY MONTHS AT THE BEGINNING AND END OF THE PROJECT

| | Referral Source | | | |
| | Police/Courts | | Other Social Agencies | |
	Before	After	Before	After
	13	40	26	23
	19	28	18	22
	24	33	14	17
	14	34	17	11
	14	22	11	12
	26	34	26	13
Total	110	191	112	98
Mean	18.33	31.83	18.67	16.33

ferrals from this source came entirely from the police alone, there is no reason to think that the increase is due to systematic increases in referrals from the court instead of from the police.

Summary

Although the sample sizes for some of the analyses presented in this chapter are necessarily small, the statistical significance of the separate results, and the consistency with which comparable results were obtained from several different sources of data, support the conclusion that the project was instrumental in effecting changes in police intervention in crisis situations. As a whole, these results indicate that the enthusiastic regard for the project expressed by the Police Department is justified.

As far as is possible, the results attest to the feasibility of approaching secondary preventive goals by improving the mental health related activities of policemen. The actual accomplishment of such a goal is finally dependent on the effectiveness of treatment intervention which follows the early case finding and management strategies implemented in this project, however. Assessment of the outcome of such efforts is an important task of community mental health, but lies outside the scope of this project. Moreover, further follow-up of the effects of this project in the future would bolster the confidence with which such efforts might be undertaken by others. However, these results in themselves should provide encouragement to those who are in a position to develop similar programs. While such projects will generate considerable work for clinician and researcher alike, policemen across the country are already engaged in trying to perform these important mental health functions for better or worse.

Chapter IX

ATTITUDES

T HE THEORETICAL BASIS for influencing attitudes through the consultation project was described in Chapter III. It will be helpful to review here the place of attitudes and attitude change in psychological theories and in the overall mental health strategy of the project in order to interpret the evidence on the results of these efforts.

It has been traditional in psychology to assume that attitudes precede and effect behavior in an action sequence. This sequence is implicit in Caplan's (1970) theme interference reduction method of mental health consultation. According to this conceptualization, an attitude is a central psychological state which is one of the determinants of behavior. Frequently, social intervention programs such as this one evaluate their effects by measuring changes in attitudes (Lipsitt and Steinbrunner, 1969; Sikes and Cleveland, 1968), on the grounds that such changes are assumed to lead to changes in behavior. In attempting to change attitudes then, it is necessary to be concerned with the relationship between attitude change and its eventual aim, alteration of behavior.

A different sequential approach to attitude change is represented by cognitive dissonance theory (Festinger, 1957). It has been shown that individuals who are induced to engage in behavior which is discrepant from their attitudes under conditions of minimal reward will subsequently change their attitudes to conform to their behavior (Festinger and Carlsmith, 1959). Presumably, this attitude change would then help to maintain the behavioral change, and perhaps lead to other new behaviors.

A third possibility is to view both attitudes and behavior as responses, and to consider the relationship between them as a kind of generalization which may operate in either direction (Zimbardo

111

and Ebbesen, 1969). This social learning theory perspective would seem to be especially useful in understanding the persistence of behavioral changes across situations which may differ in stimulus conditions and reward contingencies.

The strategy of the consultation project was to attempt to change both behavior and attitudes simultaneously in an effort to generate additional changes beyond those which were taught specifically. It is to be hoped that the effects of the project would generalize not only to the policeman's everyday work behavior as was shown in Chapter VIII but to a wider range of effectiveness in a variety of situations other than those covered in training and consultation activities.

It was assumed that generalized changes in police behavior which resulted from the project would depend on changes in attitudes. In the case of crisis intervention it was felt that the tendency to regard the mentally disturbed as incomprehensible and dangerous would have to be modified to an attitude that disturbed behavior is understandable and not necessarily threatening in order for policemen to begin to make more effective, *approach* responses to disturbed behavior. It was anticipated that the exposure and contact experiences included in the project would facilitate changing the emotional component of this attitude, while the training exercises would influence cognitive components of the attitude and tie attitude changes to new behavioral responses.

Concerning interagency cooperation, it was expected that the mutual familiarization and exchange of information would result in greater agreement among the participating agencies in attitudes toward the community. Discussion of this activity in preceding chapters has already indicated some of the behavioral changes which resulted from it.

However, it is possible that behavioral changes could occur with little or no modification of attitudes, if the existing attitudes were less avoidance oriented then they were assumed to be, or if the new responses could be seen as consistent with them. Finally, it is possible that behavioral changes could occur without accompanying changes in attitudes even when attitudes are inconsistent with that behavior, if the rewards for the behavior were great enough. The cognitive dissonance effect of subsequent changes in attitudes is not expected to occur under such reward conditions. Behavioral changes obtained under these last three conditions would not be expected to generalize to other situations as widely as when attitudinal changes are achieved.

These latter possible effects could not be ruled out entirely. Behavioral changes of the kind reported in this study should be relatively easy to effect under the conditions which existed. The consultants had the clear support and sanction of key administrators in the department, and were given a legitimate role in the training program. The specific behavioral changes advocated by the consultants had behind them the weight of approval from those to whom the policemen were accountable for their behavior, and were sometimes backed up by changes in departmental policies. It would have been somewhat surprising if such changes had not occurred at all. Still, as noted earlier, rewards for police behavior in this area of activity cannot be considered either systematic or very powerful, so it is difficult to specify what the reinforcement effects might be.

On the other hand, people are not ordinarily held accountable for their attitudes except as they are expressed in behavior. It is necessary for attitudes to be expressed in order to measure them, but it is possible to reduce the connection between attitude expression and reward contingencies somewhat by obtaining anonymous attitude measures. The attitude measures themselves can assess whether or not attitude changes occurred, and the differences in the conditions under which attitudinal and behavioral responses were obtained may provide clues to the process by which changes were effected in either or both domains. In addition, by sampling attitudes related to a wider range of situations than those immediately involved in the training activities, it is possible to determine the extent to which any changes produced in these activities may generalize to other situations. To the extent that such generalization occurred, there would be reason for optimism about the long term effects of the changes on police behavior.

Method

Two attitude instruments were employed to measure attitude changes. A 72-item Mental Health Questionnaire (MHQ) was constructed by the consultant staff. The items were written to reflect community-oriented issues concerning mental health problems which the preliminary familiarization activities indicated were salient to police work. Subjects were asked to respond to each item on a five-point Likert-type scale, ranging from *strongly disagree to strongly agree*. The MHQ was administered to all commissioned personnel in the Police Department and to professional staff members of the county unit of the State Hospital and Community Mental Health/Mental Retardation Center at the beginning and end of the project. The pretest scores of the mental health personnel were used as criteria for scoring the MHQ items. Items on which the mean response of the mental health personnel was in the direction of disagreement with the statement were scored in reverse. Responses to each item were scored from zero to four, with higher scores indicating more agreement with attitudes which were endorsed by the mental health personnel. A total score was obtained by summing across items. According to this procedure, a total score on the MHQ could range from zero to 288, and a score in which the average item response was at the midpoint would be 144. The MHQ was used to measure changes in attitudes toward disturbed behavior.

The second attitude instrument was Fessler's (1952) C-Scale. This questionnaire was originally developed to assess solidarity or consensus of attitudes toward central community activities, and consists of 40 items with the same five-point response format as the MHQ. The items are scored on eight scales, reflecting attitudes towards institutionalized behavior in each area. The scales are Community Spirit, Interpersonal Relations, Family Responsibility, Schools, Churches, Economic Behavior, Local Government, and Tension Areas. The C-Scale was administered along with the MHQ, and was used to assess changes in attitudes towards the community in general.

In order to insulate the attitude scale responses from possible reward expectancies, all questionnaires were administered anonymously. Subjects were asked to identify only their organization and years of experience. This procedure created a methodological dilemma, since an individual's before and after scores could not be matched with each other and appropriate statistical methods for repeated measures could not be employed. This meant that the data for most of the analyses had to be treated as though the groups were independent, and although there was some turnover of subjects from one time to the other, the samples were not actually independent. However, the use of such a procedure generally produces more conservative results; that is, the chances of finding significant differences are somewhat reduced. This risk seemed preferrable to altering the possible reward contingencies of the attitude responses, but must be kept in mind in interpreting the data.

It was possible to compare the attitudes of new cadets who received training during the project with the attitudes of other policemen so as to have independent groups, but this design has other shortcomings which require additional assumptions.

Policemen with two years or less experience at the beginning of the project were used as a control group against which to compare the policemen who had gone through the training program. Both before and after scores were obtained for the control groups, but only post-test scores could be obtained for the new cadets, since they were not in the department at the time of pretesting. This design is comparable to Design 12c. described by Campbell and Stanley (1963), except that subjects were not assigned randomly to the respective groups. Thus, it is necessary to assume that the two groups were comparable to each other at the time they entered the police force. While this assumption is difficult to verify, the consistency of the very rigorous selection criteria and procedures applied to both groups makes it unlikely that the groups would differ significantly in their initial attitudes and personal knowledge of members of both groups did not suggest any systematic differences in this respect. Comparison of project-trainee post-test scores with control group pretest scores matches groups which are similar in length of service, but involves measures taken at different times, and variations in overall departmental attitudes across this time interval, rather than the effects of the project, might account for any differences found. Comparing project-trainees with control group post-test scores involves scores taken at the same time, but from groups who differ in length of experience, and control group scores might be subject to any pretest effects which were present. Again, these qualifications must be considered in examining the data.

Results

Mental Health Questionnaire

As would be expected, the total MHQ scores of the mental health personnel were significantly higher than the police scores both before and after the project. The respective before and after mean scores for each group were, state hospital, 216.94 and 209.14; Mental Health Center, 219.63 and 204.46; and Police Department, 171.90 and 170.56. In an analysis of variance of this data, there was a significant main effect for time across groups ($F = 7.33$; $df = 1/528$; $p < .007$). The police scores did not change significantly, and the time effect can be attributed largely to statistical regression of the relatively extreme scores of the mental health personnel.

For the project-trained policemen, the mean MHQ score did not differ significantly from the control group pretest score, but, it did differ significantly from the control group post-test score ($t = 2.30$; $df = 84$; $p < .05$). The scores for these comparisons are presented in Table V. From the data in Table V, it would seem that the comparison of project-trainees' and control group pretest scores is justifiable, since neither the control group or the total sample changed significantly in scores from one time period to the other. This comparison involves the control group assumed to be the most similar to the project-trainees, and the difference does not support a conclusion that attitudes were changed. While it is possible that the absence of changes between the before and after attitude measures from the control group and the total police sample could be due to a consistency effect resulting from pretesting, this would not influence either of the scores in the comparison of project-trainees and control group pretest scores. The fact that the second comparison reaches statistical significance can be seen to result from a slight downward shift in control group scores, possibly due to selective attrition in the questionnaire returned by that group, and this difference could be produced by pretest effects. It may also be noted that the project-trainee scores did not differ significantly from those of the total police sample. Therefore, even with the limitations of the research design, it seems safe to conclude that significant generalized attitude changes toward disturbed behavior did not occur.

It is still possible that specific attitude changes related to the training program did occur, but did not generalize sufficiently to show up in the total MHQ scores. The project-trained and control groups were compared on the basis of their scores on each item of the MHQ to determine whether some more limited attitude changes might have occurred. There were no statistically significant differences between the groups on any of the individual items, and this possibility also cannot be supported.

C-SCALE: There were significant differences between the mental health groups and the police on only two of the eight scales at the time of the pretesting. Mental Health/Mental Retardation staff scores differed significantly from police scores on the Tension Areas scale (t = 3.02; df = 260; p < .01). State Hospital staff scores on this scale were intermediate between the other two groups and not significantly different from either. Both mental health groups differed significantly from the police in scores on the Churches scale. For the Mental Health Center-Police comparison, the *t* ratio was 3.30 (df = 260; p < .01); and for the State Hospital-Police comparison it was 3.07 (df = 262; p < .01).

Analysis of variance of the before and after scores for all three groups yielded a significant interaction effect for groups and time on the Tension Areas scale (F = 3.05; df = 2/525; p < .05). The interaction effect on the Churches scale did not reach statistical significance (F = 1.67; df = 2/525; p = < .19). The difference between state hospital and police scores on the Churches scale de-

TABLES V

MEAN MHQ SCORES FOR POLICEMEN

| | Time | | | |
| | Before | | After | |
Group	n	Mean	n	Mean
Project-trained	—	—	54	171.44
Control	38	167.97	32	166.72
Total police sample	248	171.90	211	170.56

creased somewhat, but was still significant ($t = 2.24$; $df = 236$; $p < .05$). This was the only significant difference between the groups on any of the scales at the time of the second testing. The mean scores for each group on these two scales are presented in Table VI.

The C-Scale results appear to reflect the effects of the project itself rather than methodological artifacts. It is difficult to assume that the differences are the result of sampling variations or the random occurrence of significant differences among the scales, since the pattern of before and after scores is consistent with respect to scales and directions. While it is possible that the results again reflect statistical regression of extreme scores, there is evidence with respect to this data that such was not the case. The scores which shifted were not especially extreme, and scores of comparable position on the other scales did not show a similar change, which would be expected if the effect were due to regression.

The major changes occurred in the attitude scores of the mental health staff, while police attitude scores did not change significantly. Certainly, it is overly optimistic to expect changes in the overall attitude scores of the policemen, either because of the influence which those attending the meetings might have had on other policemen or by expecting any changes in attitude scores of those attending to materially influence the mean scores of such a large sample. While it was impossible to identify the scores of

TABLE VI

MEAN SUB-SCALE SCORES ON C-SCALE

| | | | *Groups* | | | |
| | *State Hospital* | | *MH/MR Center* | | *Police* | |
Scale/Time	*n**	*Mean*	*n*	*Mean*	*n*	*Mean*
Tension Areas						
Before	17	9.88	15	7.80	247	11.45
After	30	10.27	14	10.57	208	11.09
Churches						
Before	17	7.94	15	7.27	247	11.23
After	30	8.87	14	10.21	208	10.98

* The sample sizes in this analysis vary from those of the MHQ analyses because of differences in usability of answer sheets or omissions of information.

those individual policemen who attended the meetings, it was possible to select from the police group a smaller sample which was known to contain those individuals and thus improve the chances that any changes in their attitudes would be reflected in the scores for the group.

A subsample of 54 policemen who reported ten or more years of experience was selected and scores on the pre- and post-test C-Scales were compared. The mean before and after scores in this subsample differed only slightly, and insignificantly, from each other and from those of the overall police sample. Therefore, it cannot be concluded that the police attitudes changed.

It may be that due to differences in the nature of the organizations, the attitudes of the mental health groups are more free to change than those of the policemen, or that policemen as a group view their responses to an attitude questionnaire differently than do the mental health personnel, so that they feel constrained to respond more consistently. This would suggest an effect of pre-testing, rather than no effect from the project.

It is also possible that the groups may respond to influence attempts according to different time sequences. According to this view, it may be that policemen respond to such projects at the attitudinal level more slowly than at the behavioral level, and more time will be required for the behavioral effects to generalize to the attitudinal effects than was available during the span of this project. On the other hand, most police intervention projects have shown fairly immediate attitudinal responses, but these changes frequently dissipated with equal rapidity (Sacon, 1971) and do not generalize at all to behavioral changes. Sampling either behavior or attitudes at two points in time reveals nothing about the possible cyclical patterns which might be revealed by more frequent and extended sampling. From a practical standpoint, this latter procedure has much to commend it, too. Some policemen expressed dislike for the task of completing the attitude questionnaires, and others may have had similar feelings which were not expressed except as they might have been manifested in omitting such information as years of experience, failing to complete one of the questionnaires, or failing to follow directions so that a questionnaire was unusable. While such instances were in the minority, briefer more frequent attitude sampling might have resulted in an adaptation to the task so that it seemed more palatable and could have yielded more meaningful information. These organizational and temporal considerations are not mutually exclusive, and each warrants further discussion in reflecting on the implications of this experience for future attempts at intervention.

Within the limits of the available data, the possibility remains viable, at least, that the changes measured in the behavioral domain, in the form of police performance, simply do not generalize to changes in the attitudinal domain as measured in this study. This may be so either because the intervention did not produce a central psychological change which was general enough to effect responses in other domains, or because the attitude measures did not represent a class of responses sufficiently similar to those responses which did show a change, and, therefore, generalization should not have been expected. In either event, there is no evidential basis for assuming that the project changed those attitudes which were measured in such a way that one could expect more generalized behavioral changes to occur as a result of changes in these attitudes. These results do not rule out the possibility of more generalized behavioral changes, but since their occurrence cannot be anticipated on the basis of the attitudinal data, the burden of proof will have to rest on subsequent behavioral observations.

PART IV

REFLECTIONS AND PROPOSALS

Chapter X

DISCUSSION OF RESULTS

The effort really to see and really to represent is no idle business in face of the constant force that makes for muddlement.

—Henry James

THE EVIDENCE PRESENTED indicates that the consultation project did have some effects, yet it did not produce others that were expected. The task of this chapter is to examine the results in an effort to provide a better understanding of what happened, from which suggestions for future activities may be derived. This process requires a careful examination of the conditions under which effects did or did not occur.

It is clear that the Police Department values the activities which were conducted, and has been willing to provide a variety of material supports and philosophic commitments to this kind of enterprise. Moreover, the department's efforts to continue the program speak at once to its perceived value and to the increased likelihood that it will live up to its promises. One could take the cynical position that it is in the public relations interest of the department to do so, and of course, it is. But it should be pointed out that this particular police department had already included in its program a number of training activities which are not part of the preparation of police officers in many communities and the department is not vulnerable to the claim that, relative to other departments, it was not doing enough. The program was implemented under conditions which did not constitute a reaction to an immediate crisis situation, as are some such programs, and was based on deliberate examination of the problems, resources, and alternatives. Finally, it should be repeated that no media publicity was given to the project, so that the departmental reaction cannot be attributed to a concern with public images.

Gardner (1968) has pointed out that organizations in difficulty often suffer from an inability to see their problems, rather than from a lack of capacity to solve them. In this case, the department was aware of a problem and elected a course of action to solve it. From the evidence presented here, it can be concluded that this choice has produced some encouraging results, and promises to continue to do so as long as the activities are valued by the policemen and resources are available. But, as Gardner notes further in the work already cited, social programs may create other problems even while they are serving the purposes for which they were intended, and some attention to this possibility may be helpful in predicting future effects of this project.

The multiply-determined nature of any social organization dictates that its activities must be compatible with, if not in the service of, a number of purposes besides those which the activity is primarily intended to achieve. Occasionally, innovative programs become so diffuse that they fail in their main aims while reaching subsidiary goals of relatively little consequence. More often, as the main ambitions are fulfilled, new problems are created which necessitate the setting of new goals. It is possible to view this phenomenon either as an evolutionary process of social development or as an accidental blunder. The extent to which the actual occurrence of the latter can be avoided may well depend on the degree to which the former view is given self-conscious consideration in planning social innovations. It is with this perspective in mind that the effects of the consultation project can now be examined.

Attitudes and Behavior

The reader may have the impression that a great deal of attention has been paid to the issue of the relationship between attitudes and behavior in light of the limitations in the way the data were collected, and in view of results indicating that the attempts to change attitudes were apparently unsuccessful. One might be satisfied that behavioral results were obtained and let it go at that. However, to the extent that negative results can be useful in making a point, and in this case there are other positive results which help to make the point more valid, examining the relationship between attitudes and behavior may lead to some useful hypotheses which can guide future planning.

The data on family crisis intervention and referrals reflect the efforts of the entire department, and it could not be determined to what extent the cadets who were trained during the project might have contributed to the observed changes after they were commissioned. In measuring attitudes, however, it was possible to obtain data from the project trainees as well as the department as a whole, and it was expected that since relatively more efforts were made to influence attitudes through the cadet training program, attitudinal changes should show up more strongly in this less experienced subsample. Since there were no measurable attitude changes in any of the police samples, it cannot be assumed that the behavioral changes resulted from systematic changes in attitudes.

As for the behavioral changes themselves, while the proportion of personal-social interventions in family disturbance situations increased when any action was taken, the relative frequency of intervention or nonintervention in disturbances did not change. These results could imply that the policemen's predilection for intervention in general did not change, as might have been expected to follow from attitude change, and that the mere giving of information about referrals provided a substitute response which was used only when the policeman would previously have taken some other action. Providing referral information may have implied sanction for its use, but this sanction was apparently not perceived as encouragement for increased intervention in general. These changes would not necessarily require shifts in attitudes, and the fairly constant level of the proportion of cases in which action is taken probably reflects the strength of the general departmental policy of minimal intervention.

To what extent can it be expected that cognitive dissonance effects will result from this change in behavior and eventually produce changes in attitudes? It is clear that such effects have not occurred yet, and whether or not they will appear eventually is dependent on the presence of conditions of dissonance. Leaving aside for the moment questions of the influence of departmental policy and rewards, it may be that the behavioral changes observed are not dissonant with the policemen's attitudes at all.

Making a referral does not reflect a particular attitude toward disturbed behavior as much as it involves an attitude toward the appropriateness of a community resource for dealing with disturbed behavior. Policemen may refer people for mental health services out of a sympathetic desire to provide help, because they see the mental health system as a more effective means of behavioral control than the legal system for some classes of behavior, or merely as a way of passing responsibility for a difficult problem on to someone else. Merely providing information about referral sources could lead to increased referring behavior based on any of these attitudes without necessarily changing them. If making a referral satisfied any of these desires, there is no reason to expect that a situation of cognitive dissonance would exist which might produce attitude change. On the contrary, those attitudes which exist might be reinforced.

Although the consultation project was not designed to demonstrate or analyze specific questions of attitude-behavior relationships, the results reported here suggest that attitude change is not a necessary condition for achieving behavioral change. Reviews of numerous other studies on attitude-behavior congruences in regard to group prejudice (Wicker, 1969) and mental illness (Rabkin, 1972) indicate clearly that the relationship between measured attitudes and behavior is at best a modest one, and that other personal and situational variables influence behavior in ways that are at least as important as are the effects of attitudes. Furthermore, these observations would suggest that changes in behavior without changes in attitudes do not automatically create conditions favoring cognitive dissonance, and thus there is no clear basis for predicting eventual induced attitude change.

As Smith (1968) has pointed out, several different attitudes may be engaged with a particular behavior at different times, depending on how situational variables might influence either attitudes, behavior or both. It would be naive, therefore, to assume that specific attitudes and behaviors are linked to each other in a one-to-one fashion, yet such a mistaken assumption is not un-common in social intervention projects covering a wide range of social institutions and problems.

Effects of Increasing Referrals

If one assumes that the completion of the referral process leads to effective service in meeting human needs, then the policeman's attitudes may only be important insofar as they are instrumental to his making the referral and doing so effectively. Making a re-ferral to a mental health service is not inherently better than giving advice about legal recourses unless the persons being re-ferred perceive the former action as more appropriate to their needs than the latter, and the service received is effective in deal-ing with their problems. The data on the increased number of referrals made by policemen which led to contact with the Mental Health Center indicates that referral advice was given effectively when it was used. Evaluating the effectiveness of the service re-ceived goes beyond the scope of this report, of course, but to the extent that a community mental health center can, as it should, act as a broker for bringing appropriate social resources to bear on human problems, even a few inappropriate referrals may be preferable to none at all. If, by such a process, problems can be treated earlier than would otherwise have been true, and this treatment reduces the likelihood of occurrence of a more severe problem which would have been manifested later, then secondary prevention can be achieved as a result of this project with a popu-lation which might not ordinarily be reached by mental health services.

Other factors, such as departmental policies and the rewarding and constraining effects of other police experiences, are undoubt-edly more powerful in influencing police behavior than the tech-niques employed in this project. One question of concern is whether the consultative intervention might interact with these other influences to produce less desirable unforeseen effects. For example, might the reinforcing effects of increased referral be-havior lead to an excessive reliance on this response and inter-fere with employing other more appropriate alternatives? The only evidence which can be brought to bear on this question at present comes from an internal analysis of the personal-social interventions in the post-project sample, and from less systematic observations of police behavior.

Among the personal-social interventions taken by policemen, agency referral comprised only part of the responses. Policemen also engaged in more efforts to mediate disputes and to help the parties reconcile their differences. In the incident described in Chapter VII, while the policeman brought the person to the station in search of an appropriate helping resource, it was his personal manner of handling the situation which was instrumental in helping the individual regain his composure. Referral information evidently did not constrain other helping behavior in these situations, and it is possible that knowledge of referral sources and other alternatives which can be drawn upon when needed also serves to increase the policeman's confidence in his own efforts to provide help in dealing with disturbed behavior.

Since information on referral sources had been made available to policemen in at least two forms prior to the initiation of this project, and since some training in handling disturbed behavior had been provided previously by the Police Department and the Mental Health Association, none of the effects found here, including increased referrals, can be attributed entirely to the mere provision of information or to training in any form. It can be concluded that the particular combination of activities in this program was instrumental in producing these effects, but it cannot be specified that any one aspect was more influential than another. Subjectively, it was believed that each activity was necessary to accomplish particular goals, and activities were only initiated when there seemed to be a need for them which was not being met by other efforts. However, more systematic research than was possible within this project would be required to answer this question definitively. For example, in addition to the activities conducted, the continuing stimulus effect of the consultant's presence may have been an important factor in tying the effects of the project together.

It seems probable that expectations of attitude change at this stage in the project are premature, and that while the activities of the project might set the stage for eventual changes in attitudes, the efforts to increase the policeman's exposure to and contact with disturbed behavior may only result initially in a generalized increase in such behavioral contact in his everyday work. Attitude changes, if any, would then be dependent on the policeman's actual experience in dealing with such situations, and it is probable that not enough policemen have had a sufficient number of successful experiences in dealing with disturbed behavior since the beginning of the project to have produced such changes.

Before leaving the question of attitudes, it is worthwhile to reflect on the nature of the data presented here from the perspective of its limitations and implications in understanding police behavior. In discussing the attitude measures, attention has been given to the mean scores on the particular instruments employed as representative of the entire group, and this is obviously only an approximation of the true state of affairs. There are individual differences among policemen in their attitudes, and these existed both before and after the project. The scores of some individual policemen were as high as the mean scores of the mental health group, while those of others were far lower. One would expect that policemen with different initial attitudes would vary in their receptivity to learning new behaviors and in the amount of benefit they might obtain from such experiences. In this project, it was felt that initial efforts should be directed at the department as a group by placing relatively more reliance on a generalized training approach. It was assumed that this would eventually generate more requests for individual consultation in which such differences would be more salient.

Furthermore, although the MHQ was constructed to reflect those attitudes which were related to the policeman's work encounters with disturbed behavior, it is not proposed that this scale is a sufficient sample of those attitudes. The compromises which had to be made for purposes of attempting to evaluate the project limit the utility of this data for a systematic study of police attitudes as such. Additional studies of the relationship between particular attitudes and police work are worthwhile in their own right, but could also lead to improved methods of measurement and evaluation. Instead of relying on external criterion groups and instruments developed in other contexts, such studies could be done more effectively using criteria derived from the study of effective policemen and lead to the development of more appropriate instruments. It is hoped that reports such as this one can help to stimulate further systematic work on these problems.

The results of such research are not necessary, however, to draw some important implications for psycho-social intervention from the results of this project and reports of other programs which have been cited earlier. In Chapter III it was mentioned that attitude change was not a sufficient basis for inferring the achievement of successful intervention. The results reviewed here amplify the point that attitude change is not a necessary goal in order to achieve behavioral change, and certainly should not be an exclusive or perhaps even an important target of intervention. Behavioral change may be accomplished by attending to the rewarding and sustaining elements of social systems and by the definitions which policemen make of situations based on the information available to them.

Information is, of course, an important ingredient of attitudes, but the disposition of policemen to act on the information which they have may be influenced more strongly by the social norms and expected rewards emanating from their social system than by the emotional components of their personal attitudes. Under these conditions, intervention programs can increase their effectiveness by placing relatively more weight on providing information, obtaining administrative sanctions and modifying reward structures than by directing their efforts toward intraindividual change of policemen.

This is not to say that such efforts cannot be conducted within the framework of a consultative relationship. Rather it is to suggest that models of consultation need to be comprehensive enough to provide for a variety of intervention strategies which can be both appropriate to and effective with a variety of social systems and intervention goals. Continuous monitoring of results will then become increasingly important, and sensitive consultants will place relatively less reliance on supposedly *proven* methods of intervention.

A Sequential Approach to Consultation Goals

If the kinds of consultee problems enumerated by Caplan can be considered to form a hierarchy, as suggested earlier, then in retrospect it appears that this project has only initiated a process of development which will need continuing examination and modification. So far the activities have dealt mainly with problems of knowledge and skills, and less so with questions of consultee confidence and objectivity. As the activities of the project continue, it would be expected that the focus of attention would shift as more policemen become knowledgeable and skillful. They might then become more concerned with cases which present special problems for them as individuals, and consultee-centered consultation would become more appropriate. It is too early to determine systematically whether this has begun to happen. One possible indication of such a change in needs is the Police Department's request to include specific training in making referrals which provides an opportunity for policemen to refine their judgments and increase their confidence. As these needs emerge, the project will have to change its form and pursue somewhat different goals with consultees.

However, this process will also raise new issues and increase the salience of others. As policemen become more proficient in handling disturbed behavior, appropriate changes in policies, both in the department and in other agencies will be required to accommodate these changes. Making these changes will necessitate continued interagency cooperation. As the Community Agency Conference has already demonstrated its influence in changing policies regarding dispositions of suicide attempts and drug reactions, it will continue to be useful in making other policy changes.

As the overall competence in the department in managing disturbed behavioral situations increases, more attention will also be needed in regard to the police reward structure. There are a number of changes needed in factors which are probably already inhibiting more effective performance in this regard, but consideration of these factors will be important to maintaining the gains which have been made and increasing the psychological incentives for further development as well. Both the department and consultants will need to become increasingly aware of these influences.

These are complex issues, and the question of policy formation cannot be considered appropriately here except to mention its importance and suggest some of its effects. However, aspects of the police reward structure can be examined from a social-psychological standpoint, based on the experiences gained from this project, in such a way that both administrative decision-making and consultative practices may benefit. The consultants are convinced that an increased understanding of these phenomena in regard to police behavior is one of the major contributions of this project to their own experience. The topic of reward structures will be discussed in the next chapter before returning to a final review of the project and some proposals for further action.

Chapter XI

PSYCHOLOGY OF POLICE ORGANIZATION

REWARD STRUCTURE AND GROUP DYNAMICS

Habit is habit, and not to be flung out of the window by any man, but coaxed downstairs a step at a time.

—Mark Twain

IN THE PAST, behavioral scientists have tended to view police behavior as a function of intrapersonal traits; such as, authoritarianism, sadism, psychopathy.[19] These trait examples also suggest psychologists' tendency to study such behavior as though it were a clinical problem. However, recent developments in psychology in general, and the increasing contact between behavioral scientists and policemen in particular, have shown more concern with role-related organizational and social system factors in police behavior. Among these are the systems of psychological and material incentives, and the regularly occurring reinforcing effects of work experience in an organization which are designated by the term reward structure.

The general concept of reward structure in organizations has been reviewed by Katz and Kahn (1964). The discussion here will deal with the topic as it has manifested itself in the author's experiences in working as a consultant to police departments. This is done in an effort to illuminate and make specific some of the ways in which reward structures affect the behavior of members of this social institution.

---

[19] Recent findings indicate that policemen do not differ significantly from others of similar socio-economic background in authoritarianism (Niederhoffer, 1967).

Perhaps an intrapsychic view of police work has been tenable because the rewards of police work are not highly visible and their work has been generally regarded as low in status and in pay.[20] This assumption overlooks such concepts as adaptation-level (Helson, 1964), and implies that rewards can be encompassed exhaustively within the categories of pay and status or the gratification of personal, often socially undesirable, needs which could not be satisfied in other occupations or settings. Moreover, it is reasonable to argue that some behavioral traits are the result of, rather than a basis for attraction to, police work (Mann, 1971).

Another aspect of the historical view that may be a compelling reason for an intrapsychic perspective is the perception of police organizations as quasi-military in character. This concept provides a ready, but perhaps too facile, complementarity to such time-honored subjects of study in psychology as needs for order, conformity, and, of course, authoritarianism. There are some important differences, however, in the implications of the term military for the *real* military and the police organization, such as in the observance and legal status of limits on fraternization and discrimination by rank, and the separation of career tracks for officers and enlisted men in the armed services. Perhaps a better term for the police is semi-military, or better, hierarchical. In any case, this comparison is worth pursuing further from the standpoint of its organizational implications alone.

Incentives and Rewards

The military aspects of police organization are indeed authentic; that is to say, real; but they are not sufficient to explain police behavior or police department operations entirely. One important element of a reward-structure is promotion and advancement. Here, police departments differ from the military in several important respects.

The promotional capability of a police department is typically dependent on position vacancies, and there is a definite fixed correspondence between rank, pay and position. In the military, the

---

[20] This view has not been correct at all times in history. See Niederhoffer (1967) and Marx (1970).

rank of a person filling a particular slot may vary across several grades, promotions are based on time-in-grade and supervisor-initiated efficiency reports, and persons given a rank higher than that authorized for their position can be transferred laterally to another organization. Moreover, since the minimum 20-year retirement option in the military probably creates more turnover at the top than is true in police departments, the military would seem to enjoy an advantage in both position openings and promotional capacity. Thus, a police department's ability to provide positive incentives such as promotions is dependent on the uncontrollable occurrence of vacancies. On the other hand, promotions must occur when vacancies occur whether or not there is a deserving candidate. Even assuming that there is always a deserving candidate, this form of reward is quite remote from any specific job performance.

In addition, the promotional machinery of a police department is typically tied to a civil service system wherein written examinations are given much higher weightings than are supervisor's evaluations. The consequences of this arrangement are that promotions probably reward intelligence primarily and not necessarily competent performance. Thus, the supervisor is left with little reward power for his subordinates and probably little incentive for providing supervision except for preventing gross violations of policy or incompetent performance through the imposition of negative sanctions; e.g., reprimand, suspension.

Other consequences follow. An organization with limited positive reward power may also be inclined to minimize the tendency to employ negative sanctions as a means of maintaining organizational balance and minimizing organizational strain. Individuals can help to maintain this system if supervisors are not informed of any more than is necessary (cf. Bittner, 1970). Given limited opportunities for advancement, this system virtually assures that there will be a high attrition rate of competent people at the lower ranks. The more competent an individual, the more likely he is to have alternative job opportunities available to him outside the department. While some of the more competent will be rewarded, the others may encounter frustration and the psychological incentives for leaving the department would be increased (Thibaut and Kelley, 1959). This situation would tend to make persistence in police work less a function of high competence than of dedication and group identification. Within these limitations, what is rewarded? Although it has been estimated that no more than 20 percent of a policeman's work involves detecting and apprehending criminals, and that the remainder is spent in providing service and assistance with various human problems (Bard, 1968), virtually 100 percent of the rewards are assigned according to the policeman's record in dealing with criminal activity.

Thus, an officer who may have saved lives through a successful family disturbance intervention, an officer who may have prevented a racial disturbance because he regularly socializes with and befriends minority group youth, or an officer who understandingly and patiently prevents a suicide through sympathetic listening to a person's troubles, may be rated as substandard if his record does not reflect a sufficient number of arrests and summonses. It may be *all in a day's work,* but it is not all in another day's pay. Usually a police department does not have an adequate reporting and accounting system for these acts of quiet human heroism, which speaks of their general valuation in police work and makes systematic reward for their performance all the more unlikely.

This system of limited tangible rewards and selective partial reinforcement tends to generate a strong group dynamic in which a policeman who intends to remain on the job must seek his rewards and guide his behavior on the basis of the group cohesiveness and the social norms which that group creates. These forces are probably the strongest ones regulating police behavior and deserve careful examination.

Group Dynamics

In work with police departments, some persistent and interesting phenomena of police group behavior have been observed from which inferences about group dynamics can be drawn. In the light of the previous discussion, it can be assumed that these processes will continue to influence a policeman's behavior when he is not in the immediate physical presence of his peers.

It is helpful in understanding the background of these processes to make comparisons with the behavior of workers who share similar conditions of socioeconomic status and organization of labor (Lipset, 1969; Sterling and Watson, 1970). Thus, the tendency for policemen to have primarily other policemen as social acquaintances is understood better as a characteristic shared with other workers whose labor is organized into shift work than as a result of any personal propensity for aloofness or clannishness, or because of defensiveness (see Westley, 1970). Similarly, it has been observed that many policemen are personally somewhat shy and hesitant in relating to persons of different socioeconomic status, but this behavior is not characteristic of their other relationships.

These forces at once tend to reduce the policeman's contacts as an autonomous participant in the on-going norm-generating social processes in the larger community, to create ambiguity for them about behavioral norms which are prevalent in the community, and to necessarily force the policeman to rely on social and behavioral prescriptions emanating from his own peer group and from the rights and obligations associated with his social position as a policeman. The same forces can be said to effect any other community member who shares similar degrees of limited social out-group contact and a specialized in-group system of rewards and sanctions.

The creation and reinforcement of these group processes appear to operate most strongly on two occasions. One is during the assembly period at the beginning of each shift; the other occurs during spontaneous gatherings of police officers following an incident of an especially dangerous or emotionally arousing nature.

During the assembly period at the beginning of a shift there is a phenomenon which can best be labelled as a warm-up process. There is consistently an amount of good-natured horseplay and needling which takes place during these sessions which serve as a preliminary to the shift. During this time announcements are made to the patrolmen, the sergeants read off special notices of stolen cars, missing persons, escapees, and wanted subjects. Assignments to special details or to particular vehicles are made, notices of court appearances are passed on, and other official business is taken care of in this 15-minute period. The joshing and sharp but good-natured kidding that goes on during these sessions suggest that they also serve a very important psychological function.

Policemen live other roles in their lives as individual human beings, and they are coming from those roles into their police roles for eight hours, despite the fact that technically policemen are on duty 24 hours a day. To the extent that police work involves different attitudes and philosophies about life and about one's own behavior than do their other roles, these sessions help in making the transition.

Among the purposes served by these sessions, the following would seem to be included. First, the good humor and mutual needling seems to serve the purpose of group cohesion, since this process communicates to the participants that they are part of the group. One wonders, then about those few officers who do not participate in these activities and their relationship to the group. It may be that those officers who do not participate would also perform differently in the field than those who do. It is noticeable that there is probably less mutual horseplay between persons who differ in their length of service in the department. Those who are older participate in the warm-up activities less than those who are relatively new to the force.

A second important function of the warm-up is that it serves to discharge tension and hostility in a humorous way. This can be seen as a response to the uncertainty of what the policeman may encounter in the ensuing shift and the very real possibility of encountering violence and hostility. By trying out a kind of one-upmanship with each other during this period, the policemen prepare themselves to face challenging encounters with citizens of the community. Perhaps the discharge of hostility through needling serves to help the officer to keep these impulses under control when he is actually encountering a subject in the course of work.

A parallel phenomenon occurs at the end of a shift or following emotionally charged events such as armed robberies and high-speed chases. This may be termed a *cooling-off* process, but it, too, serves some important psychological functions.

At the termination of a work shift, police officers reassemble informally to turn in citations for the supervisor's approval and to complete and file reports. The level of discussion can best be described as loose, since many of the officers are fatigued, and there are frequent expressions of disgust or amazement at their experiences during the shift. This process is more animated following specific emotionally-laden experiences. The officers exchange their observations of the event and openly express their feelings and opinions about it. Those involved in the event describe their reactions and those not involved directly suggest how they believe they would behave under similar circumstances. The author has described elsewhere (Mann, 1971) how this post-crisis emotional comparison process can be influential in establishing group norms. In general, these cooling off sessions serve to relieve some of the frustration-induced anger and resentment which the policeman might build up during his shift on duty.

Another important function of the cooling-off session is that it serves to bring the officers back together once more after they have been relatively isolated on patrol during the shift. This serves to renew group ties before going off duty, and to reassert the importance of group membership. Further testimony to the importance of this effect is a monthly party which is held by the members of the evening shift at the time shift assignments change. Since they will be changing to day-time assignments, there is a longer than usual time between work shifts, and this party serves both as a celebration and an affirmation of group spirit.

Another group dynamic influence has been observed in the course of efforts to establish consultation relationships with field supervisors, who hold the rank of sergeant. It was comparatively easy to consult with the supervisory personnel at the level of captain and lieutenant, and with the young patrolmen and cadets. However, repeated difficulty was encountered in attempting to establish contact with the sergeants. In general, they were the least well informed about the purposes of consultation, and efforts to schedule training sessions with them to develop relationships were consistently delayed.

The sergeants appear to be key figures in efforts to help policemen in handling disturbed behavior in the community because of the potential influence they could exert over patrolmen. On the basis of theory and previous research they were not expected to be the most inaccessible group (Mann, 1972), and this phenomenon demanded further study.

In an effort to better understand this problem several key personnel were interviewed with reference to this occurrence. By and large, the information obtained did not provide answers which were entirely satisfactory. The most frequent response obtained was that there was no real problem except difficulties of scheduling. However, using this information as a starting point, clues to some aspects of this phenomenon may be suggested.

The patrol activities of the police department may be viewed organizationally as one of the most insulated segments of police activity relative to outside innovations. There are real reasons for this state of affairs in the form of relatively little face-to-face contact with peers, maximal spatial dispersion of activities, and a high degree of individual discretion in decision-making compared to other police activities. Bittner (1970) has analyzed these factors in detail. As primary supervisors of this activity, the patrol sergeants would seem to exercise considerable relative autonomy within the department.

While it is true that finding free time for scheduling training sessions with these supervisors could be a problem, few people in the department acknowledged that this was a significant factor. It seems more meaningful to view this phenomenon in the dynamic terms of a power-dependency relationship, such as the model suggested by Dalton, Barnes and Zaleznik (1968).

Some interviewees felt that maintenance of control over field supervisors by command level officers (lieutenants and captains) was an important domain of influence. If, as the analysis presented here suggests, this control is tenuous, then it makes sense that its maintenance would be closely guarded. Command level supervisors can ill afford to have their immediate subordinates acquire skills over which they themselves do not feel a sense of mastery, because the legitimacy of their assessments of performance and administration of rewards in this area might be questioned. Since most of the command level supervisors' reward power lies in approval or disapproval of the arrest behavior of the patrols, by determining whether or not a booking will be made, the expansion of subordinates' competencies into areas not under this kind of control can be expected to be viewed with circumspection. It can be hypothesized that this tendency may be exaggerated when the power-dependency relationship is based on a limited range of rewards which can only partially influence subordinate behavior.

On the other hand, since the approval or disapproval of arrest behavior is a key factor in the policeman's role as it is typically defined, this aspect of reward structure is a powerful influence over the field supervisors. It is understandable that they may complement the viewpoint of the command supervisors by restricting their own role commitments to behaviors which fall within the domain to which rewards can be applied.

Another factor in the relative inaccessibility of the uniformed sergeants as a group may be a degree of competition between the different shifts, the organizational element with which they are most closely identified. Evaluations of shift performance are made in part on a comparative basis and there is some intershift social comparison which is generated by this process. This state of affairs could serve as a barrier to bringing the field supervisors together as a group, but it is probably of secondary importance to the factors involved in the command-field supervisors relationships.

The failure to anticipate these occurrences was due partly to incomplete understanding of how the theory should be applied to the particulars of the police department. A formal analysis of the organizational structure of the department would suggest that lower ranking personnel should be more accessible to innovation, based on the assumption that lower status is associated with weaker ties to central authority. While it is questionable whether this assumption holds for police organization, a more *functional* analysis of police organization would have highlighted the relative autonomy of the field supervisors and their mutual interdependence with the command level supervisors, which can now be described from hindsight. It is worth noting that this interdependence is heavily supported by the internal police norms about what constitutes proper (rewardable) police behavior.

This analysis of reward structure can contribute more than merely to qualify the limitations on introducing innovations in police work. It can point out why a training program may be difficult to implement, but it can also illuminate why training alone is insufficient and suggest other required modes of change.

In essence, this analysis indicates that in order for a change in police behavior to endure, the resultant changes in role relations must be given official as well as unofficial legitimacy, not merely through public pronouncement, but by establishing a record keeping system which will reflect the changed behavior and by making provisions for rewarding such behavior within the role of the policeman, rather than in an *ad hoc* fashion, such as through occasional citations of merit. Additionally, both supervisors and consultants could make more deliberate use of the normally occurring social comparison processes to establish changes in mutual expectations and self-evaluations. In turn, such processes could improve supervisory practices and, potentially, overall police effectiveness. This informal kind of in-service training may ultimately be more effective than several varieties of classroom sessions.

It must be recognized that policemen already perform a broad range of activities, only some of which are officially designated as part of the policeman's role. In reality, these tasks are of at least equal importance to the community as those which are publicly recognized. But the enormity of the task of redefining and achieving normative support for changes in role designations cannot be taken lightly. Already this debate has reached the level of several Presidential commissions, and the issues are far from being settled. The point of these remarks is that while social-psychological understanding of police reward structure and the development of innovative techniques are helpful and necessary, the redefinition and recognition of police role functions is a product of social forces larger than a consultation program or a police department. It is properly the result of a community process of debate, goal-setting, and decision-making, and while one sees all too little of the last two parts of this process on the contemporary scene, increased police competence and appropriate rewards for performance are one means of initiating such a process.

Even within current conditions in most communities, there is enough freedom to change that the observations presented here could be implemented to a degree large enough to be beneficial. It is not being suggested that social psychological knowledge will solve problems by itself, but competent police administrators are making increasing use of knowledge from this field and others in trying to deal with problems which require all the knowledge which can be brought to bear on them. Further studies of these processes can surely be beneficial. To recall Gardner's (1968) observation, it may be that the hardest part of the task will be to recognize the need.

Chapter XII

SUMMARY AND RECOMMENDATIONS

While men believe in the infinite, some ponds will be thought to be bottomless.

—Thoreau

THE PSYCHOLOGICAL consultation project has served a number of goals. It has served as a means of demonstrating a form of co-operative enterprise between psychologists and policemen, it has shown that new ways of meeting the mental health needs of a community can be generated effectively, and it has provided an opportunity to explore the efficacy of a variety of psycho-social intervention techniques. However, it has also been very much a *learn-while-doing* kind of activity, and this aspect of the process would not be complete without attempting to integrate the experiences, lessons, and effects into a systematic framework which can serve as a guide to improving future efforts of a similar nature.

It should not be assumed that this or any other demonstration can serve as an exact blueprint to guide such activities. Although it is possible to assert some principles of psycho-social intervention, a more important contribution is to raise questions about procedures which are assumed to be an established part of conventional wisdom, and generate a process for considering alternatives. While an outline or model can aid in considering problems of consultation and social change systematically, it must be recognized that the choice of goals to be achieved and the methods for pursuing them are partially dependent on the characteristics of particular social systems.

Participation in Planning and Goal Setting

In recent years it has become increasingly prevalent that people pay attention to the process of planning, and systems for allocating resources toward goals have been developed and popularized most notably because of the success which the space program has had with such procedures. However, an important step which is not provided for explicitly in such systems is occasionally overlooked when applying them to other problems. This is the process by which goals are established and the participation of relevant groups in their selection.

The presence or absence of shared goals has been cited as an important ingredient of the consultation process (Glidewell, 1959), and while many social programs have suffered from a lack of agreement on goals, little has been presented to guide the process of goal selection. Often the establishment of goals is viewed as a political, that is to say, competitive, process in which the goals of one party are assumed to be inherently in conflict with those of another. While this may often be a realistic appraisal of the situation, the mistake lies in failing to question this assumption and in not exploring the possibilities of finding areas where there are shared goals or reconciling the conflicts among goals through discussion.

It is doubtful that the psychological consultation project could have achieved much if it had not begun with a discussion of goals in which several elements of the Police Department participated. Not only did this serve to initiate the project with the cooperation of key personnel, but it also served as a continuing reference point against which progress could be reviewed by both policemen and consultants. This informal contract of goals, which is more than a contract for services, provided a basis for discussing problems encountered and for considering changes in methods and strategies which is indispensable to the kind of in-process modifications that are needed to allow such projects to adapt to changing situations.

Thus, there are two important dimensions to the goal-setting process which have important functional implications for the conduct of psycho-social intervention programs. One is the extent to which goals are shared between consultants and the consultee system, and the other is the breadth, one might say the diffusion, of the sharing of those goals within the consultee system itself. As only one example of how these elements may affect a consultation program, the author has reported elsewhere (1972) how a lack of breadth in the sharing of consultative goals within a consultee system can interact with social-psychological characteristics to create differential accessibility of members of the system to the consultant. An extremely dramatic example of conflicting goals as an impediment to progress in a consultation program is described by Glidewell and Stringer (1967).

Monitoring of Processes

Once a basis for periodic review of progress has been established by the selection of goals, intervention programs require continuous information which can indicate the need for such review and can suggest the focus of changes which might be considered. This was done rather informally in this project through frequent and regular interviews with key personnel, attendance at the preshift briefings, and through feedback obtained in consultations. However, it would seem desirable to establish a more systematic monitoring process which could provide information for both evaluation and planning.

At the beginning of this report, it was noted that an important and often neglected aspect of evaluation is to collect and examine evidence on the process of innovation as distinct from the outcome. This procedure involves the collection of data relevant to the allocation of resources, the achievement of intermediate goals, and the modification of programmatic elements in keeping with the planned strategy of innovation. While the information presented here is insufficient for a formal systems analysis of such a program, the data can be regarded in a process analysis framework so as to provide examples of the kinds of information which might be collected and the types of questions which might be addressed to the data.

A further possibility is to view the observations presented here as a source of information about the processes involved from which more formalized procedures of program implementation and systems analysis might be developed. Using such a perspective, it is possible to consider choices among alternatives for the direction of future efforts.

According to this frame of reference, the project has served to clarify the way in which psychological goals related to attitude change, behavioral change, and the transfer of training and consultation experience to work settings might be ordered into hierarchies of intervention goals so as to be more feasible and effective. While attitude change may be where the action is for some psychologists, it is clear that information, new ways of behaving, and testing out techniques and procedures in actual experience is more nearly in line with the kinds of expectations for change which policemen hold. When the process is viewed in this latter perspective, it can be concluded that the intermediate goal of changing police intervention in crises has been accomplished, and that now more attention should be focused on the remaining elements of the secondary preventive process. In turn, the accomplishment of this intermediate goal has changed some of our assumptions about what is necessary to achieve these changes.

Further analysis of the effects of the project, based on data not presently available, would be required to determine if the shift in strategy in the program, in which it was decided to give more attention to problems of knowledge and skill, will eventually lead to more problems of confidence and objectivity being presented in response to opportunities for individual case consultation. Such data would provide a test of the hierarchical notion of consultee problems as well as to serve a monitoring function from which future changes in consultative activities could be planned.

From the standpoint of resource allocation, it can be seen that the Police Department has contributed significantly to the conduct of the program so far by engaging in cooperative planning, by providing guidance, suggestions, and feedback, by making time and personnel available in the various training activities, and by sanctioning their conduct. At the same time, there is no reason to change the conceptualization of the field supervisors as key figures in building the change of mental health functions into operational patterns within the department. Making these personnel available for training sessions is a key resource allocation which has not yet occurred. A second concern of this kind is the allocation of resources in the form of rewarding police behavior in this area, which has already been discussed. A third question in this domain is the provision of funding for the continuation of further activities. At the present time, financial support for future activities has tentatively been promised, but if the program is to become truly a part of the department's activities, either the funding should come directly through the city budget, or the continuing relationship between the department and outside funding sources will need to be formalized with an eye towards continuity.

Furthermore, as the project continues, there will be a natural tendency for it to spread into other activities and to be picked up for implementation in other settings. Again, this process requires careful analysis of the problems involved, the resources available, and the kinds of strategies required to apply the resources to the problems effectively. Care will be required to insure that adequate resources are available to meet emerging new concerns without sacrificing the quality of current activities which need to be continued. As additional programs may be stimulated by this one, attention will need to be given to the selection of problems which can be solved with the resources available, and which can potentially result in the development of new, additional resources for program development.

It can be concluded that programs such as the one reported here can be effective in improving the mental health functions of policemen, functions which they are already performing. Moreover, the improvement in the delivery of mental health services, the reduction of potential hazards to policeman and citizen alike, and the ultimate improvement in the quality of community life which can result from such actions can be accomplished with relatively little cost. Hopefully, as these efforts continue, increased knowledge of community processes and understanding of human behavior can contribute to the solution of a widening range of social problems.

At the same time, there are limits to the transferability of social innovations to different settings. Other innovative programs have previously demonstrated some of the concrete effects reported here in improving police management of crisis situations (Bard, 1970) and promoting increased interagency cooperation (Rhodes, *et al.*, 1968). In one sense, this project served to replicate those demonstrations, but in another sense it was the aim of this project to create a broad-based change in the relationships of social institutions to each other and to their clients that would develop as a program which belonged to the participants rather than to a group of experts, and would continue to grow beyond the demonstration period. The evidence which can be gathered on this latter aim at this time is limited but encouraging. Furthermore, special care has been taken to describe each element of the program in detail as regards the conditions under which the work was done, the interpretations given to these conditions, and the strategies that were implemented in response to them, so that others who wish to conduct similar activities can benefit from this experience. To further this end, some words of caution are in order.

Replicability of Demonstration Projects

The history of demonstration projects suggests that transferring activities conducted in one situation to another is frequently unsuccessful. Where this failure occurs, it should be obvious that some critical ingredients have been omitted. While some elements of demonstration projects may be difficult to replicate, such as the enthusiasm of the participants for a novel activity, or the unique abilities of a particular set of individuals (subjects as well as agents of the program), it is equally likely that transfer fails because the same conditions were assumed to exist when in fact they did not.

One element of this program which cannot be emphasized too strongly is the relationship which was developed between the consultants and the police. It is nearly a law of social action that relationships are the things on which programs ride. It should be clear by now that it is more than just the personal character of relationships which is helpful, although that aspect is critically important. It is the sense of mutual participation in the definition of problems, planning, and cooperative implementation which is the real moving force behind action programs. In observing this rule, it follows that such programs will operate with the existing social system, its norms and expectations, rather than against it, and this will necessarily affect the form of the program. But it seems unlikely that efforts which attempt to do otherwise will have much survival value.

A second important program element is that the innovation

must be tailored to fit the needs and resources of the particular organization and community, taking into account the regularized operational patterns, structures, and functions of each as well as their problem. Here also, the relationships described above are of critical value. It is doubtful that much progress could have been made in this project without the continual participation in planning and review sessions of members of the Police Department.

To the extent that one can generalize about policemen, we found them to be extremely knowledgeable about the dynamics and problems of their own social system and the kinds of techniques required to effect change. More than once their pragmatic attitudes forced us to reexamine and concretize some of our theoretical thinking so that in the end we both understood the situation more clearly.

Whether or not the same kinds of activities can be effective in achieving these goals in other communities will depend on their appropriateness to the particular police department, community, and problems under consideration. One example of such a consideration has been cited already in comparing the strategy of this project, in a medium-sized city, to that conducted by Bard and his associates (1970) in New York (see Chapter III). But even in other comparable communities, important differences may exist in political conditions, the history of police department relationships to other similar *outsiders,* the problems which exist in mental health service delivery, and many other factors. It is hoped that those elements of this project which are useful to such endeavors will be more likely to be employed because of this report, that those which are inappropriate will be discarded, and, to paraphrase an old prayer, that the reader will have the wisdom to know, or seek, the difference.

Mental Health Implications

When the delivery of mental health services is viewed as a social system process, the police can be seen to constitute one element among many which are linked together. The activities reported here serve to highlight and increase recognition of the police role in this system, but this is only one aspect of the larger process. As the police function in this system improves, it is necessary also to attend to the other parts of the system. This need was implicitly recognized in the establishment of the Community Agency Conference in this project, and the conference, or a similar vehicle, may contribute to growth and improvement of the total service delivery system.

In this context, it is also important to note the limitations on what kinds of goals can be accomplished through this type of intervention. The project activities are relevant to goals of secondary prevention in a community mental health framework, and can enhance the accomplishment of that goal by intervention in behavioral crises, sometimes to the end of resolving the crisis in the direction of growth for the participants, but more often by initiating a process which may include for the subjects in crisis increased self-examination, utilization of community services or other social resources, and a change in the equilibrium of the family system which triggers the crisis. Thus, the action of the police can set in motion personal and social forces which may in the end improve the mental health of persons who might otherwise suffer a decrement in effective living, but the actual realization of that goal will depend in many instances on factors which the policeman does not control. For example, increasing referrals to an already overburdened mental health delivery system could possibly decrease the effectiveness of the entire system, and where inadequate or no services exist, more of the burden for secondary prevention would fall on the policemen themselves as mental health agents, and would require a dramatic redefinition of the policeman's role and of the consultative functions.

To the extent that the lives of children affected by these crisis situations can be improved by effective crisis intervention, some progress could potentially be made toward goals of primary prevention, although those goals can probably be pursued more effectively by other means. In general, the Police Department as a social institution is not in an advantageous position to pursue activities relevant to primary prevention. Just as Bittner (1970) notes that the police can do little to reduce crime because they do not control the causes of crime, so it is with mental health problems. Much of police activity is organized to be reactive to citizen-definition of specific problem situations within a wider range of potential problem incidents. Among those events about which policemen receive complaints, their actions are determined to some extent by the definition of the problem by complainants, rather than the existence of a problem in some absolute sense (see Black and Reiss, 1970).

Effective Community Functioning

If mental health is defined broadly as an attribute of the quality of life in a community, then it is possible to conceive of the police as having an important, though still only a partial, role in primary enhancement of positive mental health. When the concept of police-community relations comes to be regarded as placing more emphasis on community relations in a positive sense, and not just as a means of resolving or controlling problems between policemen and citizens, then an appropriate vehicle for the primary prevention of problems of community life would be at hand. Some relatively new programs in a few cities have such a potential, but their success will depend on a change in the definition of the police function from one of social control to one of social enhancement, on the one hand, and on the extent to which other elements of the community system will shoulder their share of the burden rather than relying heavily on the police to assume most of the responsibility.

Where such changes occur, it is more likely to be a function of the philosophy, organization, and involvement of the community itself, and not just the police department. Among the changes which will have to occur is an end to the traditional isolation of policemen from larger social interaction. As mentioned earlier, this will require greater familiarity of policemen with more of the detailed characteristics of community life. It will also depend on greater familiarity of citizens with policemen.

Until the exact form of the future is more clear, it can best be approached in a spirit of cooperative problem solving and shared anticipation. Whatever the route that is taken, the journey will be easier if some of the unneeded, excess ideological and social baggage can be intelligently discarded at critical choice points on the road to community development.

BIBLIOGRAPHY

Albee, G. W.: *Mental Health Manpower Trends*. New York, Basic Books, 1959.

Bailey, W. D.: Family Disturbances. Unpublished paper, Criminal Justice Project. University of Texas School of Law, Austin, Texas, 1970.

Bard, M.: Alternatives to Traditional Law Enforcement. Paper presented at American Psychological Association. Washington, D.C., September, 1969.

Bard, M.: Family Intervention Police Teams as a Community Mental Health Resource. *Journal of Criminal Law, Criminology and Police Science,* 60:247-250, 1969A.

Bard, M.: Extending Psychology's Impact Through Existing Community Institutions. *American Psychologist,* 24:610-612, 1969B.

Bard, M.: *Training Police as Specialists in Family Crisis Intervention.* Washington, D.C., U.S. Department of Justice, 1970.

Bard, M.: and Berkowitz, B.: Training Police as Specialists in Family Crisis Intervention: A Community Psychology Action Project. *Community Mental Health Journal,* 3:315-317, 1967.

Bennis, W. G.: *Changing Organizations.* New York, McGraw-Hill, 1966.

Berscheid, E. and Walster, E. H.: *Interpersonal Attraction.* Reading, Mass., Addison-Wesley, 1969.

Bittner, E.: *The Functions of the Police in Modern Society.* Chevy Chase, Md., National Institute of Mental Health, 1970.

Black, D. J. and Reiss, A. J.: Police Control of Juveniles. *American Sociological Review,* 35:63-77, 1970.

Brown, B. S.: Philosophy and Scope of Extended Clinical Activities. In C. F. Mitchell (Ed.) : *Extending Clinic Services into the Community.* Austin, Texas, Texas State Department of Health, 1961, pp. 5-9.

Caplan, G.: *Prevention of Mental Disorders in Children.* New York, Basic Books, 1961.

Caplan, G.: *Principles of Preventive Psychiatry.* New York, Basic Books, 1964.

Caplan, G.: The Nature and Problems of Evaluation in Community Mental Health. In Leigh M. Roberts, N. S. Greenfield and M. H. Miller (Eds.) : *Comprehensive Mental Health: The Challenge of Evaluation.* Madison, Wis., University of Wisconsin Press, 1968, pp. 3-14.

Caplan, G.: *The Theory and Practice of Mental Health Consultation.* New York, Basic Books, 1970.

Cowen, E. L., Gardner, E. A. and Zax, M. (Eds.) : *Emergent Approaches to Mental Health Problems.* New York, Appleton-Century-Crofts, 1967.

Cumming, E., Cumming, I. and Edell, L.: Policeman as Philosopher, Guide, and Friend. *Social Problems,* 12:276-286, 1965.

Dalton, G. W., Barnes, L. B. and Zaleznik, A.: *The Distribution of Authority in Formal Organizations.* Boston, Harvard University Press, 1968.

Fessler, D. R.: The Development of a Scale for Measuring Community Solidarity. *Rural Sociology,* 17:144-152, 1952.

Festinger, L.: *A Theory of Cognitive Dissonance.* Evanston, Ill., Row, Peterson, 1957.

Festinger, L. and Carlsmith, J. M.: Cognitive Consequences of Forced Compliance. *Journal of Abnormal and Social Psychology,* 58:203-211, 1959.

French, J. R. P. and Raven, B.: The Bases of Power. In D. Cartwright (Ed.) : *Studies in Social Power.* Ann Arbor, Mich., Institute for Social Research, University of Michigan, 1959, pp. 150-167.

Fried, M.: Evaluation and the Relativity of Reality. In L. M. Roberts, N. S. Greenfield and M. H. Miller (Eds.) : *Comprehensive Mental Health: The Challenge of Evaluation.* Madison, Wis., University of Wisconsin Press, 1968, pp. 41-78.

Gans, H. J.: *The Urban Villagers.* New York, The Free Press, 1962.

Gardner, J. W.: *No Easy Victories.* New York, Harper and Row, 1968.

Gibb, J. and Lippitt, R. (Eds.) : Consulting with Groups and Organizations. *Journal of Social Issues,* 15: No. 2, 1959.

Glidewell, J.: The Entry Problem in Consultation. In J. Gibb and R. Lippitt (Eds.) : Consulting with Groups and Organizations. *Journal of Social Issues,* 15:No. 2, 51-59, 1959.

Glidewell, J. C. and Stringer, L. A.: The Educational Institution and the Health Institution. In E. M. Bower and W. G. Hollister (Eds.) : *Behavioral Science Frontiers in Education.* New York, Wiley, 1967, pp. 384-400.

Goffman, E.: The Insanity of Place. *Psychiatry,* 32:357-388, 1969.

Gurin, G., Veroff, J. and Feld, S.: *Americans View Their Mental Health.* New York, Basic Books, 1960.

Helson, H.: *Adaptation-Level Theory.* New York, Harper and Row, 1964.

Hollingshead, A. B. and Redlich, F. C.: *Social Class and Mental Illness.* New York, Wiley, 1958.

Joint Commission on Mental Illness and Health: *Action for Mental Health.* New York, Basic Books, 1961.

Katz, D. and Kahn, R.: *The Social Psychology of Organizations.* New York, Wiley, 1964.

Kelly, J. G.: The Mental Health Agent in the Urban Community. In L. J. Duhl (Ed.) : *Urban America and the Planning of Mental Health Services.* New York, Group for the Advancement of Psychiatry, 1964, pp. 474-494.

Lewin, K.: *Field Theory in Social Science.* New York, Harper and Row, 1951.

Liberman, R.: Police as a Community Mental Health Resource. *Community Mental Health Journal,* 5:111-120, 1969.

Lipset, S. M.: Why Cops Hate Liberals—and Vice Versa. *Atlantic Monthly,* 223: No. 3, 76-83, 1969.

Lipsitt, P. D. and Steinbruner, M.: An Experiment in Police-Community Relations: A Small Group Approach. *Community Mental Health Journal,* 5:172-179, 1969.

Mann, P. A.: Police Responses to a Course in Psychology. *Crime and Delinquency,* 16:403-408, 1970.

Mann, P. A.: Establishing a Mental Health Consultation Program with a Police Department. *Community Mental Health Journal,* 7:118-126, 1971.

Mann, P. A.: Accessibility and Organizational Power in the Entry Phase of Mental Health Consultation. *Journal of Consulting and Clinical Psychology,* 38:215-218, 1972.

Mann, P. A. and Iscoe, I.: Mass Behavior and Community Organization: Reflections on a Peaceful Demonstration. *American Psychologist,* 26:108-113, 1971.

Mannino, F. V. and Shore, M. F.: *Consultation Research.* Washington, D.C., U.S. Department of Health, Education and Welfare, Public Health Monograph, No. 79, 1971.

Marx, G.: Civil Disorder and the Agents of Social Control. *Journal of Social Issues,* 26:19-57, 1970.

Maslow, A. H.: A Theory of Human Motivation. *Psychological Review,* 50:370-376, 1943.

Matthews, R. A. and Rowland, L. W.: *How to Recognize and Handle Abnormal People.* New York, National Association for Mental Health Inc., 1964.

Newman, R. G. and Keith, M. M. (Eds.) : *The School-Centered Life Space Interview.* Washington, D.C., Washington School of Psychiatry, 1964.

Niederhoffer, A.: *Behind the Shield.* Garden City, N.Y., Doubleday and Co., 1967.

Pettigrew, T.: Racially Separate or Together? *Journal of Social Issues,* 25:43-69, 1969.

President's Commission on Law Enforcement and Administration of Justice: *Task Force Report: The Police.* Washington, D.C., U.S. Government Printing Office, 1967.

Rabkin, J. G.: Opinions About Mental Illness: A Review of the Literature. *Psychological Bulletin,* 77:153-171, 1972.

Rapoport, L.: The State of Crisis: Some Theoretical Considerations. *The Social Science Review,* 36: No. 22, 1962.

Rhead, C., Abrams, A., Trossman, H. and Margolis, P.: The Psychological Assessment of Police Candidates. *American Journal of Psychiatry,* 124:11, 1575-80, May, 1968.

Rhodes, W. C.: *Training in Community Mental Health Consultation in the Schools.* Chicago, American Psychological Association, 1960.

Rhodes, W. C., Seeman, J., Spielberger, C. D. and Stepbach, R. F.: The Multiproblem Neighborhood Project. *Community Mental Health Journal,* 4:3-12, 1968.

Rhodes, W. C.: Community Structures for the Regulation of Human Behavior. In S. Golann and C. Eisdorfer (Eds.) : *Handbook of Community Psychology and Mental Health* (in Press).

Sacon, S.: *An Intensive Training Program for a Police Department.* Washington, D.C., American Psychological Association, September, 1971.

Schulberg, H. C., Sheldon, A. and Baker, F. (Eds.): *Program Evaluation in the Health Fields.* New York, Behavioral Publications, 1969.

Seashore, C. and Van Egmond, E.: The Consultant-Trainer Role in Working Directly with a Total Staff. In J. Gibb and R. Lippitt (Eds.) : Consulting with Groups and Organizations. *Journal of Social Issues,* 15: No. 2, 36-42, 1959.

Sherif, M.: Superordinate Goals in the Reduction of Intergroup Conflict. *American Journal of Sociology,* 63:349-358, 1958.

Sikes, M. and Cleveland, S.: Human Relations Training for Police and Community. *American Psychologist,* 23:766-769, 1968.

Smith, M. B.: A Map for the Analysis of Personality and Politics. *Journal of Social Issues,* 24:No. 3, 15-28, 1968.

Sofer, C.: *The Organization from Within.* Chicago, Quadrangle Books, 1961.

Sterling, J. and Watson, N. S.: Changes in Role Concepts of Police Officers. *Mental Health Program Reports,* No. 4. Bethesda, Md., National Institute of Mental Health, Publication No. 5026, 1970.

Thibaut, J. W. and Kelley, H. H.: *The Social Psychology of Groups.* New York, Wiley, 1959.

Westley, W. A.: *Violence and the Police: A Sociological Study of Law, Custom and Morality.* Cambridge, Mass., MIT Press, 1970.

Wheeler, L.: *Interpersonal Influence.* Boston, Mass., Allyn and Bacon, 1970.

Wicker, A. W.: Attitudes versus Actions: The Relationship of Verbal and Overt Behavioral Responses to Attitude Objects. *Journal of Social Issues,* 25: No. 4, 41-78, 1969.

Zajonc, R. B.: The Attitudinal Effects of Mere Exposure. *Journal of Personality and Social Psychology Monograph Supplement,* 9:2, Part 2, 1968.

Zimbardo, P. and Ebbesen, E. B.: *Influencing Attitudes and Changing Behavior.* Reading, Mass., Addison-Wesley, 1969.

COMMUNITY AGENCY CONFERENCE PARTICIPANTS

Austin Independent School District
Austin Police Department
Austin-Travis County Community Mental Health/Mental Re-
  tardation Center
Children's Unit, Austin State Hospital
Crisis Telephone Service
Human Opportunities Corporation
Travis County Juvenile Court
Travis County Unit, Austin State Hospital
University of Texas Police Department

Appendix II

MENTAL HEALTH QUESTIONNAIRE

Directions: For each item in this questionnaire, you are to indicate the degree to which you agree or disagree with the item. You have the following choices:

1. Strongly Disagree
2. Somewhat Disagree
3. Neutral
4. Somewhat Agree
5. Strongly Agree

Make no marks on the questionnaire. Use the special answer sheet.

You should blacken the space between the lines on the answer sheet corresponding to your choice for each item. Please answer all items. Be sure you blacken the space for your choice completely with the special pencil given you. Make only one choice for each item. If you wish to change an answer, be sure to erase the first mark completely. Check occasionally that you are marking for the number on the answer sheet which corresponds to the item number on the questionnaire.

1. The present *lunacy* laws provide clear-cut guidelines for efficient handling of these cases.
2. Improving the underlying economic and social problems in a community would probably reduce the incidence of mental health problems.
3. Mental disturbance is a medical problem and has little to do with the way a person lives.
4. People whose behavior is disturbing to others usually have some kind of mental problem.
5. It is important for one social agency to be able to handle all the problems of any particular client.
6. If a person is disturbed enough to be placed in a mental hospital, then he should be kept there behind locked doors so that he cannot just simply walk off the grounds.

158

7. There is little or no friction between the police department and other agencies involved in mental health concerns.
8. Psychiatrists should be empowered to make people stay in treatment until the psychiatrist decides the person should be released.
9. One has a duty to stop a suicide from occurring if at all possible.
10. People should not try to be helpful to mentally disturbed people unless they are qualified professionals in a mental health specialty.
11. Family disturbances should be handled through a show of force.
12. The concept of mental health means the same thing to rich people as it does to poor people.
13. Probably the best way to avoid trouble in dealing with a mentally disturbed person is to be very direct and show your authority, so that they understand that you are completely in control of the situation.
14. The disposition of mental health cases is very efficient at this time.
15. Any person, no matter how mentally disturbed, must still be held to be responsible for his actions.
16. Many suicide attempts may be viewed as an asking for help by a very unhappy person, as opposed to a genuine attempt to kill oneself.
17. Some agency other than the police department should assume responsibility for the lonely old ladies who repeatedly call the department for reassurance and attention.
18. It would be a good idea to have a county-wide register of social agency cases so that any agency could know who is being served by other agencies.
19. Most mentally disturbed people would be able to get along better in the community if people were more tolerant of them.
20. Every person who might be suspected of being mentally disturbed and who has been placed in jail should be interviewed by a psychiatrist.
21. Policemen handling family disturbances should try to pro-

vide whatever help they can, even if no law has been broken.

22. Mental institutions discharge people before they are ready to return to society.

23. After a person has been treated for a mental disorder and released from treatment, it is unlikely that the person will have further difficulty with that problem.

24. The ordinary citizen is not capable of helping mentally disturbed people.

25. Once a person has been admitted to a mental institution, he should become the institution's responsibility, even if he escapes.

26. Most *normal* people could develop psychopathological symptoms under stressful conditions.

27. Social class influences the type of treatment one receives for mental problems.

28. Most police officers are skilled in dealing with mentally disturbed persons.

29. Anyone who attempts suicide is obviously severely mentally disturbed and should be placed in a mental hospital for a period of time.

30. People have no business expecting policemen to help them with their personal problems.

31. Alcoholics Anonymous probably does a better job of dealing with alcoholics than any other single agency.

32. Cooperation between law enforcement agencies and social agencies in handling disturbed persons is about as good as can be expected.

33. People with many different kinds of problems should be in contact with the social agencies which can provide specialized service for each kind of problem.

34. It is appropriate for policemen to take initial responsibility for mental health problems arising within the context of their work role.

35. Mentally disturbed persons make unreliable employees.

36. To the extent that policemen engage in *caregiving* activities their police enforcement role suffers.

37. Most nonprofessional people will only harm the mentally disturbed person by trying to help him.
38. Mentally disturbed persons are not responsible for their own behavior.
39. Drunks aren't really different from alcoholics. Both words refer to people who drink too much alcohol.
40. A mentally disturbed person should always be handcuffed while being taken into custody since they may become violent at any moment.
41. Most mentally retarded persons need to be cared for in special institutions.
42. The police work role is not well understood by the other agencies in town.
43. Psychologically sophisticated policemen tend to be good policemen.
44. State hospitals should have a maximum security area for criminal patients.
45. Communities are usually prepared to accept chronic mental patients who are released after being in a mental hospital for many years.
46. Early detection of mental illness doesn't really do that much good, since most mental illnesses can't be treated anyway.
47. Women seem to have many more mental problems than men.
48. Suicidal individuals do not usually hint to others that they intend to kill themselves.
49. It is very important that people who show signs of mental disturbance receive psychiatric treatment as soon as possible.
50. Patients who have spent many years in a mental hospital are usually eager to be released.
51. When intervening in a family fight, it does little good to try to determine who was at fault, since blaming someone will just increase his hostility.
52. Well-intentioned efforts by persons without professional mental health training to help the mentally disturbed only delay their receiving proper treatment.
53. Most patients in mental hospitals are dangerous.

54. It is important that mentally disturbed people be removed from the situation they are in until they can recover from their condition.
55. The community mental health center should coordinate community interventions in mental health situations.
56. Family quarrels are often dangerous and should be handled by policemen.
57. The need to protect professional confidences make it impossible for social agencies to share information about clients with each other.
58. Most mentally disturbed people receive more sympathy than is good for them.
59. Most policemen consider taking escaped mental patients back to state hospitals a nuisance.
60. Family disturbances are potentially dangerous situations.
61. There should be some other agency in a community for handling drunks and alcoholics other than the police.
62. Hospitalized mental patients should be allowed to work in the community under supervision.
63. Recurrent family disturbances cannot be prevented.
64. Sometimes older people who live alone begin to act strangely largely because they have so little contact with other people.
65. Proper disposition of *lunacy* cases requires full cooperation between the state hospital and the police department.
66. Police are often called into family quarrels only as a last resort.
67. Policemen should receive greater training in dealing with community mental health problems.
68. Most mentally disturbed people show rapid fluctuation of mood, and thus are highly unpredictable.
69. The presence of a policeman tends to have a calming effect on family disturbances.
70. Once an alcoholic always an alcoholic.
71. Policemen play a minor role in coping with community mental health problems.
72. Policemen should be able to call on trained mental health personnel for help in dealing with disturbed persons.

INDEX